MRCGP PRACTICE EXAMS

SECOND EDITION

MRCGP PRACTICE EXAMS

SECOND EDITION

JOHN E. SANDARS MB ChB (Hons) MRCP (UK) MRCGP
Examiner, Royal College of General Practitioners.

REBECCA BARON MB ChB DRCOG MRCGP
GP and Vocational Training Course Organiser, Stockport, Cheshire.

PASTEST
KNUTSFORD
CHESHIRE

First printed in 1985
Reprinted 1987
Revised Edition 1989
Second Edition 1992

A catalogue record for this book is available from the British Library.

ISBN 0-906896-92-4

Text prepared by Turner Associates, Congleton, Cheshire
Printed in Great Britain by Dotesios Ltd.

CONTENTS

INTRODUCTION TO THE MRCGP EXAM

The number of candidates sitting the MRCGP examination each year is now over two thousand. Although, at approximately 70%, the overall pass rate is higher than that of other postgraduate medical exams, the MRCGP exam cannot be described as easy and should not be taken lightly. Examination fees mean that failure is expensive.

The examination is set by the college as an 'assessment of the knowledge, skills and attitudes appropriate to the general practitioner on completion of vocational training, assessing the competence of candidates to carry out unsupervised responsibility for the care of patients in general practice'.

The exam syllabus covers a great breadth of knowledge and the exam itself aims to measure knowledge, skills and attitudes within the five areas of general practice.

1. Clinical Practice — Health and Disease
2. Clinical Practice — Human Development
3. Clinical Practice — Human Behaviour
4. Medicine and Society
5. The Practice

The syllabus is shown in detail in the RCGP publication *The Future General Practitioner — Learning and Teaching*, available direct from the Royal College of General Practitioners, 14 Princes Gate, Hyde Park, London SW7 1PU.

The object of taking the MRCGP examination is to become a member of the College. There is no other way of becoming a member at the present time.

Eligibility — usually any doctor who is eligible for the Joint Committee for Postgraduate Training in General Practice (JCPTGP) certificate is eligible to take the MRCGP examination. If there are any doubts then you should apply to the Membership Secretary at the Royal College. At present, pre-certification in cardiopulmonary resuscitation and child health surveillance is required. The exact requirements are subject to change and the current requirements will be sent to all applicants for the examination.

Applications - the examination takes place twice a year, usually mid May and late October/early November. The closing date for applications is about eight weeks before the exam. The written papers can be taken in several centres but oral examinations are held only in Edinburgh and London.

Format - There are five parts to the exam, each of equal value. Although each part counts for 20% of the final total it is not necessary to pass each individual part, since a good performance in one part can compensate for a poorer performance in another.

The three written papers are taken on one day and the two orals are taken on another day about six weeks later.

Three Written Papers:
>   The Multiple Choice Question Paper (MCQ) — 2 hours
>   The Modified Essay Question Paper   (MEQ) — 2 hours
>   The Critical Reading Question Paper (CRQ) — 2 hours 15 minutes

Two Orals:
>   Oral 1 : Practice Experience Questionnaire — 30 minutes
>   Oral 2 : Topics not covered in the first oral — 30 minutes

The three written papers are marked first, the marks are then added together and averaged and then candidates are divided into three groups:
1.   Candidates whose average mark is above the pass rate are invited to attend the oral exam. Usually 50% fall into this group.
2.   The intermediate group of candidates are also invited to attend the oral exam. They may be able to pass the exam overall if they do well in the orals despite a borderline fail on the written papers.
3.   The clear fail group (approximately 15%) who do so badly in the written papers that they have no chance of passing the exam and are not invited to attend the orals.

Thus approximately 85% are invited to proceed to the orals.

The theory behind the examination
An examination sets out to test what has been learnt during a period of study. It is not easy to set a good exam, especially in the field of medicine, where not only knowledge but also skills and attitudes are being assessed. A good

examination needs to be valid and reliable. Valid in that the desired educational objectives are efficiently assessed, and reliable in that these objectives are measured with consistency. The Royal College has gone to great lengths to construct a valid and reliable exam despite the difficulties of trying to measure knowledge, skills **and** attitudes. The examination has been subject to research by the Centre for Medical Education of the University of Dundee and has developed under their guidance. No other postgraduate medical exam has been so carefully evaluated. An excellent description of the background to the exam can be found in Occasional Paper Number 46: *The MRCGP Examination* edited by Cameron Lockie, available from the Royal College of General Practitioners.

The Written Papers.
> MCQ. Knowledge is measured. Performance in this part is a good predictor of overall examination performance.

> **MEQ and Critical Reading Paper.** Skills of interpretation and problem solving are tested. In addition there is some attempt to identify and evaluate the candidate's attitude to various problems.

The Orals.
> These assess knowledge, skills and attitudes with particular emphasis on the latter.

The exam is constantly being evaluated and modified in the hope of keeping abreast of changing public and professional needs. Currently, there is debate as to whether it should become the accepted standard of training for new principals. This would then require the development of an alternative method of assessment for established principals. At the moment, due to demands from the public and within the profession, a form of clinical assessment is planned placing emphasis on the central importance of the consultation (and the attendant communication skills required) in general practice.

Who Fails?
It is important to remember that illegibility can be a reason for failure. If your answer cannot be read, it cannot be marked! The written word as an effective method of communication is vital. Failure to answer the question

asked, either because of poor time organisation or misinterpretation of what is being asked, also results in low marks.

Candidates appear to perform badly in the following areas due to lack of knowledge:
  Social and legal medicine
  Practice organisation (including organisation of NHS and FHSA)
  Natural history of disease and epidemiology
  Cardiology
  Dermatology
  Therapeutics (especially drug interactions and side effects)
  Obstetrics and Family Planning
  Ophthalmology
  Paediatrics

Poor marks in the MEQ and Orals are often due to:
  Paucity of ideas
  Not considering a sufficient number of options
  Inability to justify options
  Inability to organise thoughts leading to rambling answers

Attitudes are difficult to assess but failure in the orals can be caused by several attitudes which examiners find unacceptable:
  An authoritarian and inflexible doctor-centred approach to solving the patients' problems.
  Failure to recognise patients' rights such as autonomy.
  Lack of ethical consideration in the area of confidentiality.
  Lack of an understanding of the importance of continuing education as shown by lack of critical reading.

THE FIVE AREAS OF GENERAL PRACTICE

The MRCGP exam syllabus covers a great breadth of knowledge and the exam itself aims to measure knowledge, skills and attitudes within the Five Areas of General Practice.

1. Clinical practice — Health and disease.

The candidate will be required to demonstrate knowledge of the diagnosis, management and, where appropriate, the prevention of diseases of importance in general practice. This area includes:

    a. The range of normal
    b. The patterns of illness
    c. The natural history of diseases
    d. Prevention
    e. Early diagnosis
    f. Diagnostic methods and techniques
    g. Management and treatment

2. Clinical practice — Human development.

The candidate will be expected to possess knowledge of human development and be able to demonstrate the value of this knowledge in the diagnosis and management of patients in general practice. This area includes:

    a. Genetics
    b. Foetal development
    c. Physical development in childhood, maturity and ageing
    d. Intellectual development in childhood, maturity and ageing
    e. Emotional development in childhood, maturity and ageing
    f. The range of the normal

3. Clinical practice — Human behaviour.

The candidate must demonstrate an understanding of human behaviour particularly as it affects the presentation and management of disease. This area includes:

    a. Behaviour presenting to the general practitioner
    b. Behaviour in interpersonal relationships

    c. Behaviour of the family
    d. Behaviour in the doctor-patient relationship

4. Medicine and society.

The candidate must be familiar with the common sociological and epidemiological concepts and their relevance to medical care and must be able to demonstrate knowledge of the organisation of medical and related services in the United Kingdom and abroad. This area includes:

    a. Sociological aspects of health and illness
    b. The uses of epidemiology
    c. The organisation of medical care in the UK - comparisons with other countries
    d. The relationship of medical services to other institutions of society

5. The practice.

The candidate must demonstrate a knowledge of practice organisation and administration and must be able to critically discuss recent developments in the evolution of general practice. This area includes:

    a. Practice management
    b. The team
    c. Financial matters
    d. Premises and equipment
    e. Medical records
    f. Medico-legal matters
    g. Research

The examination is designed to assess in a variety of ways the skills of the candidate:

In interpersonal communication
In history taking, information gathering and recording information
In assessing and defining the problems presented
In making a supposition as a basis for further action (hypothesis formation)
In defining available options

In selecting examinations using investigations and procedures
In selecting therapy
In providing continuing care
In interventive and preventive medicine in relation to:
    (a) the patient
    (b) the family
    (c) the community
In the organisation of practice and self
In teamwork, delegation and in relating to other colleagues

The candidate will be expected to demonstrate appropriate attitudes to his patients, his colleagues and to the role of the general practitioner. He must demonstrate his ability to develop and extend his knowledge and skills through continuing education.

A planned approach to revision is the key to getting through the MRCGP exam.

The most important point to remember is that this is an exam about **current General Practice** and your reading needs to reflect this. Subjects such as General Medicine, Obstetrics, Paediatrics etc are included but they only make up a small proportion. In order to put this in perspective, it is helpful to look carefully at the Five Areas of General Practice on the preceding pages. You can see from this that:

Area 1: Health and Disease encompasses most of the areas covered in finals and found in textbooks.

Area 2: Human Development covers Paediatrics but also includes knowledge of the elderly.

Area 3: Human Behaviour is an important area in general practice. It covers such areas as: why patients present, consultation models, the doctor-patient relationship and interpersonal relationships as they affect patients, their families and us.

Area 4: Medicine and Society covers the epidemiology and sociology of health care e.g. knowledge of the cause of disease (for example cholesterol and CHD risk). This is vital to our methods of treating such disease. This area includes the organisation of health care — a subject that has been affecting all of us recently.

Area 5: The Practice.
This includes knowledge of practice management e.g. finances, records, premises etc. It also includes general management skills such as delegation, time management, team development.

Covering all these areas in your revision will give you the broad knowledge-base required for the exam and for life as a GP (which is, of course, what the exam was designed to do!).

At first glance, the amount of work required can seem immense but by working through the different areas logically you will see that you already have a lot of the knowledge required. Revision needs to be designed to fill the gaps. You won't fail for not understanding the cost-rent scheme (although you should know how to find out about it). You may however be on shaky ground if you know nothing about the management of a practice.

It is also important to remember that the exam reflects current practice and current research, not out-of-date books.

Bearing all this in mind, how can you start to cover the material?

Textbooks

You may need to read selected textbooks to cover areas in which your knowledge is deficient e.g. on the doctor-patient relationship or practice management. If you feel that you are lacking in basic medical knowledge, it may be worth reading a textbook but bear in mind all the other areas of knowledge as well. It is worth reading something on the common diseases in general practice.

Journals

These cover the current research in general practice. The British Journal of General Practice and BMJ are essential reading, preferably for the12-18 months up to the exam. (Remember the written exam is set in March.) This task may seem daunting — but is actually very interesting! You don't need to read everything. It is worth keeping notes on what you have read as it is useful to be able to review them near to the exam. Look especially for review articles and recurrent 'topical' themes.

Other journals such as Update, Horizons and Monitor are worth perusing as they often contain subjects not covered elsewhere, but be selective. Beware the common fault of reading articles on subjects you already know well.

Occasional Papers and Reports from General Practice

These are the current literature of general practice and hence include some vital reading. There are many available but a list is included of the most important. It is worth being aware of recent publications as these are often clues for current areas of importance in general practice.

As the amount of work can seem daunting, the best approach is to divide up the list between a group of people and ask each person to produce a short summary (i.e. 1-3 typed A4 sheets) on the paper or report which can then be shared.

Current affairs

Newspapers, television and radio will keep you up to date and aware of current issues. The media often present subjects from a different perspective which can be useful.

Hot topics

Most of these have been around for some time and again it is a matter of broad reading and being aware of current initiatives to make sure of covering them. A checklist is included to make sure you have not missed any major areas.

Planning

Go through the 'five areas' and the list of revision topics to identify a list of areas on which you want to concentrate. Start with those areas you know nothing about and, if there is time, come back to topics you know better. That way you will ensure a broad knowledge base.

Ideally, get together with other people taking the exam and share out topics and Occasional Papers to produce short summaries of each. When you read a topic, try and think about the sort of questions you could be asked e.g. managing a diabetic who will not accept his disease. Always think about the ethical issues. Remember, the difficult problems that arise in surgery are often the same ones that appear in the exam.

Practising

Practising the different components of the exam will improve your technique and help identify weak areas of knowledge. Practicing MCQs, MEQs and Critical Reading Questions is more fun in a group.

Doing, discussing and communicating are as important as sitting in a room reading.

Have an overall plan. Keep records of what you read as this helps revision and allows you to see progress from your efforts.

Steady reading throughout the year is better than pre-exam panic.

Good luck!

ACKNOWLEDGEMENTS
The practice papers presented in this book have all been extensively tried and tested by groups of MRCGP candidates. We would like to extend our warmest thanks to Dr Susan Glicher, Dr Peter Elliot and Dr Tom Boyd whose help and advice with this book have been invaluable.

It is helpful to produce your own Revision Checklist. The list will vary for each person, but should be open to addition as topical areas arise. You may like to produce a list for a group of people taking the exam and share out the topics to produce a set of summaries. In devising your list, review the Five Areas of General Practice to make sure you cover them all. You will find some areas are well known to you and can be left off your list whilst others require more work. For topics such as 'Cholesterol' there is currently research being carried out and it is useful to have a list of the up to date views on the subject. This will be of particular use in the Critical Reading Question Paper : Question 2. The following list covers most of the important area:

Hypertension
Cholesterol
Risks and benefits of the oral contraceptive pill and HRT
Terminal care
Depression
Osteoporosis
Management of common conditions e.g. sore throat, ear infections, UTI
Sexual abuse
Alcohol and drug abuse
AIDS
GP obstetrics
Resuscitation
Screening: children, adults, elderly, breast, cervical etc
Paediatric surveillance
Consultation - structure, length etc
Counselling
Doctor-Patient relationship
Effects of social class on illness
Patients' rights and complaints procedures
Patient participation
Sick doctors
Coping with your own anger and stress
Audit
Structure of the NHS
Role of the practice nurse
Computerisation
The contract and future changes
Reaccreditation tests for GPs

RECOMMENDED READING

This choice is designed to supplement your basic knowledge. It covers common areas in which candidates perform badly.

Balint M. **The Doctor, his Patient and the Illness.** 2nd edition, Pitman 1964, reprinted 1992.

British National Formulary. BMA and Pharmaceutical Society.

DHSS Publications:
Drug Tariff
Handbook of Contraceptive Services
Immunisation against Infectious Diseases
Medical Evidence for Social Security Purposes

Fry J. **Common Diseases: The Nature, Incidence and Care.** MTP Press 4th edition 1985, reprinted 1987.

Jones R.V. et al. **Running a Practice.** 3rd edition, Chapman & Hall, 1985 reprinted 1989.

Neighbour R. **The Inner Consultation.** MTP Press 1987, reprinted 1992.

Palmer K T. **Notes for the MRCGP.** 2nd edition 1992. Blackwell Scientific Publications.

Pendleton D et al. **The Consultation: An Approach to Learning and Teaching.** Oxford Medical Publications, 1984 reprinted 1991.

Pritchard P and Low K. **Management in General Practice.** Oxford Medical Publications 1989.

Statement of Fees and Allowances (The Red Book). From FHSA.

RCGP Occasional Papers and Other Publications for Summary

This list gives an idea of important papers and reports. It is important to check the full list of publications from the College sales office to look for more recent publications on relevant topics.

Occasional Papers

15 The Measurement of the Quality of General Practitioner Care (1981)
19 Inner Cities (1982)
20 Medical Audit in General Practice (1982)
22 Promoting Prevention (1983)
25 Social Class and Health Status: Inequality or Difference (1984)
31 Booking for Maternity Care: A Comparison of Two Systems (1985)
35 Preventive Care of the Elderly: A Review of Current Developments (1987)
36 The Presentation of Depression: Current Approaches (1987)
37 The Work of Counsellors in General Practice (1988)
39 Practice Assessment and Quality of Care (1988)
41 Practice Activity Analysis (1988)
43 Community Hospitals — Preparing for the Future (1990)

Reports from General Practice

18-21 Combined Reports on Prevention (1984)
22 Healthier Children — Thinking Prevention (1982 reprinted 1984)
23 What Sort of Doctor? (1985)
24 Alcohol — A Balanced View (1986)

Books and Booklets

In Pursuit of Quality (1986)
To Heal or to Harm, The Prevention of Somatic Fixation in General Practice (1987)

THE MULTIPLE CHOICE QUESTION PAPER

The MCQ paper covers the factual clinical areas in the exam. There is evidence that MCQs not only test factual knowledge but also reasoning ability and understanding of basic facts, principles and concepts. The MCQ mark for any candidate is the best predictor of his final mark in the exam. It is also the most reliable section of the exam, which means that if the candidate were to take the exam at a later date, he would tend to achieve a similar position in the ranking of candidates. The MCQ paper is set by 6 examiners, each examiner taking responsibility for 2 or 3 sections of the exam. All new questions are reviewed and modified by the whole group.

The paper will consist of questions of the true/false type, with a total of 360 questions. Stems may have a variable number of questions attached.

A mark will be awarded for each question correctly answered as true or false. Marks will not be deducted for incorrect answers or for failure to answer. You should therefore attempt all the questions. This method of marking is in keeping with current educational opinion. It seems to be a more accurate way of discriminating between candidates.

The breakdown of the questions into topics is approximately as listed below:

Medicine	60
Therapeutics	36
Psychiatry	36
Obstetrics/gynaecology	36
Paediatrics	30
Dermatology	24
Practice organisation	24
Surgical diagnosis	18
Physical medicine/trauma	18
Ophthalmology	18
Infectious diseases	12
Care of the elderly	12
ENT	12
Ethical & legal	12
Epidemiology/research	12
TOTAL	**360**

Revision

It would be comforting to read and learn a range of text books, and feel confident in answering most of the questions. This is however not advisable for a number of reasons. It would be extremely time consuming, especially if it were in place of other more relevant reading. It would not help greatly in other sections of the exam. Factual information is well covered in finals and much of the other information should be naturally acquired in practice. This is not like the MRCP and the minutiae are not what is required.

Several methods may help you improve your scoring.

- Practice as many MCQs as possible. Several books of MCQs have been produced (see Recommended Reading) and MCQs are given in a number of the magazines and journals.
- Bear in mind the topic distribution.
- Questions on practice organisation are becoming increasingly common so make sure you are up to date.
- Consider revising a little on drug interactions and child development which are easily covered and often asked.
- It is a useful exercise to try writing an MCQ yourself — you will then realise that it is not as easy as it may seem to find suitable topics!

Answering technique

Carefully read the stem with each of its following questions individually in order to be clear about the question asked. Each stem and item make up a statement which you have to mark as 'True' or 'False'. Look only at a single statement when answering, disregard all the other statements presented. Your response should be shown by filling in the lozenge on the answer sheet. It may sound obvious but it is vital to ensure the correct lozenges are filled in. The sheets are marked by computer, so if you inadvertently fill in the wrong line of answers, you could score very badly. If you wish to change an answer your mark should be erased as fully as possible and the new answer entered.

Certain trigger words are used in MCQ questions, and it is important to be clear of their meaning.

Always: Without a single exception.

Never: Not on one single occasion.
Both of these are usually false, as clinical medicine is rarely absolute — but there are exceptions!

The majority: At least 50%.

Usually: In at least half of the cases.

A characteristic feature: Occurs with sufficient frequency to be of diagnostic significance e.g. bleeding in ulcerative colitis. If the feature was absent you might doubt the diagnosis.

A typical feature: This is very similar to a characteristic feature — you would expect it to be present.

A recognised feature: A reported feature that you might reasonably be expected to know, e.g. Necrobiosis lipoidica diabeticorum — mentioned in the text books frequently — but not common or characteristic.

Is associated with: Similar to above — you should have heard of it, but it may not be common.

In 30% of cases: A given figure allows some leeway, so the figure is either approximately true or far out.

Having read the question you are faced with three possibilities:

1. **You can answer the question.** Good. Answer as you think best. Bear in mind you may still be wrong. In order to make the exam as good a discriminator as possible, questions which everyone answers correctly may be removed from the final marking.

2. **You are not sure of the answer but can use your knowledge and reasoning to work out an answer.** Many of the questions will fall into this category and you may well be able to work out the correct answer.

3. **You have no idea what the answer is.** Because you do not lose a mark for a wrong answer — guess. The removal of negative marking seems a big relief. In fact, everyone has the same advantage. With the negative marking system it was found that the more questions people answered the better they scored, so with the removal of negative marking the people likely to benefit are those who were loathe to guess.

It is worth working through the paper, answering those questions you are fairly certain about and then going back to any questions you wish to think about again. Repeatedly going over questions you have answered can be counter-productive, as answers which you were originally confident were correct may appear rather less convincing at a second, third or fourth perusal. In this situation, first thoughts are usually best. Remember the examiners are not trying to trick you — they just need to find out what you know! Don't try to look for hidden meanings, catches and ambiguities.

Most people find the exam difficult. In 1989 the mean score was 50.52% — so an average candidate is likely to perceive a large number of the questions as difficult. The minimum mark was 11% and the maximum 70%. This was before the removal of negative marking. Hence people may now score higher, but the final analysis is how you compare with your peers.

Undoubtedly some people find MCQs easier than others. You can only do your best. If you find this part of the exam difficult, then practice more MCQs to improve your technique.

Summary

1. Read each question carefully and be sure that you understand it.

2. Mark your responses clearly, correctly and accurately.

3. Use reasoning to work out the answers and guess at those you do not know.

4. The best way to obtain a good mark is to have as wide a knowledge as possible of the topics being tested in the exam.

MCQ INSTRUCTIONS

In order to help MRCGP candidates revise for this examination we have tried to follow as closely as possible the content and new format of the official examination. Each question has an answer and teaching explanation which should provide a good basis for successful revision.

We suggest that you work through this set of multiple choice questions as though it were a real examination. In other words plan to take this practice exam at a time when you will be undisturbed for a minimum of 2 hours and do not obtain help from books, notes or other people while working. Choose a well-lit location free from distractions, keep your desk clear of other books or papers, have a clock or watch clearly visible with a rubber and 2 well sharpened grade B pencils to hand.

As you work through each question in this book be sure to mark a tick or cross against each question, thus when you have completed the paper you can mark your own answers with the help of the answers and explanations given at the end of the book. Do not be tempted to look at the questions before sitting down to take the test as this will not then represent a mock examination.

The Royal College of General Practitioners

☞ Each of the 360 items on the question paper is either true or false. If you believe that the answer is true, you should fill in the T lozenge; if you believe that it is false, fill in the F lozenge. Fill in the lozenge as shown above.

☞ Enter your answers to items 1 to 150 on this side; then turn over and continue entering your answers to items 151 to 360 on the other side.

1 ⓣ ⓕ	31 ⓣ ⓕ	61 ⓣ ⓕ	91 ⓣ ⓕ	121 ⓣ ⓕ
2 ⓣ ⓕ	32 ⓣ ⓕ	62 ⓣ ⓕ	92 ⓣ ⓕ	122 ⓣ ⓕ
3 ⓣ ⓕ	33 ⓣ ⓕ	63 ⓣ ⓕ	93 ⓣ ⓕ	123 ⓣ ⓕ
4 ⓣ ⓕ	34 ⓣ ⓕ	64 ⓣ ⓕ	94 ⓣ ⓕ	124 ⓣ ⓕ
5 ⓣ ⓕ	35 ⓣ ⓕ	65 ⓣ ⓕ	95 ⓣ ⓕ	125 ⓣ ⓕ
6 ⓣ ⓕ	36 ⓣ ⓕ	66 ⓣ ⓕ	96 ⓣ ⓕ	126 ⓣ ⓕ
7 ⓣ ⓕ	37 ⓣ ⓕ	67 ⓣ ⓕ	97 ⓣ ⓕ	127 ⓣ ⓕ
8 ⓣ ⓕ	38 ⓣ ⓕ	68 ⓣ ⓕ	98 ⓣ ⓕ	128 ⓣ ⓕ
9 ⓣ ⓕ	39 ⓣ ⓕ	69 ⓣ ⓕ	99 ⓣ ⓕ	129 ⓣ ⓕ
10 ⓣ ⓕ	40 ⓣ ⓕ	70 ⓣ ⓕ	100 ⓣ ⓕ	130 ⓣ ⓕ
11 ⓣ ⓕ	41 ⓣ ⓕ	71 ⓣ ⓕ	101 ⓣ ⓕ	131 ⓣ ⓕ
12 ⓣ ⓕ	42 ⓣ ⓕ	72 ⓣ ⓕ	102 ⓣ ⓕ	132 ⓣ ⓕ
13 ⓣ ⓕ	43 ⓣ ⓕ	73 ⓣ ⓕ	103 ⓣ ⓕ	133 ⓣ ⓕ
14 ⓣ ⓕ	44 ⓣ ⓕ	74 ⓣ ⓕ	104 ⓣ ⓕ	134 ⓣ ⓕ
15 ⓣ ⓕ	45 ⓣ ⓕ	75 ⓣ ⓕ	105 ⓣ ⓕ	135 ⓣ ⓕ
16 ⓣ ⓕ	46 ⓣ ⓕ	76 ⓣ ⓕ	106 ⓣ ⓕ	136 ⓣ ⓕ
17 ⓣ ⓕ	47 ⓣ ⓕ	77 ⓣ ⓕ	107 ⓣ ⓕ	137 ⓣ ⓕ
18 ⓣ ⓕ	48 ⓣ ⓕ	78 ⓣ ⓕ	108 ⓣ ⓕ	138 ⓣ ⓕ
19 ⓣ ⓕ	49 ⓣ ⓕ	79 ⓣ ⓕ	109 ⓣ ⓕ	139 ⓣ ⓕ
20 ⓣ ⓕ	50 ⓣ ⓕ	80 ⓣ ⓕ	110 ⓣ ⓕ	140 ⓣ ⓕ
21 ⓣ ⓕ	51 ⓣ ⓕ	81 ⓣ ⓕ	111 ⓣ ⓕ	141 ⓣ ⓕ
22 ⓣ ⓕ	52 ⓣ ⓕ	82 ⓣ ⓕ	112 ⓣ ⓕ	142 ⓣ ⓕ
23 ⓣ ⓕ	53 ⓣ ⓕ	83 ⓣ ⓕ	113 ⓣ ⓕ	143 ⓣ ⓕ
24 ⓣ ⓕ	54 ⓣ ⓕ	84 ⓣ ⓕ	114 ⓣ ⓕ	144 ⓣ ⓕ
25 ⓣ ⓕ	55 ⓣ ⓕ	85 ⓣ ⓕ	115 ⓣ ⓕ	145 ⓣ ⓕ
26 ⓣ ⓕ	56 ⓣ ⓕ	86 ⓣ ⓕ	116 ⓣ ⓕ	146 ⓣ ⓕ
27 ⓣ ⓕ	57 ⓣ ⓕ	87 ⓣ ⓕ	117 ⓣ ⓕ	147 ⓣ ⓕ
28 ⓣ ⓕ	58 ⓣ ⓕ	88 ⓣ ⓕ	118 ⓣ ⓕ	148 ⓣ ⓕ
29 ⓣ ⓕ	59 ⓣ ⓕ	89 ⓣ ⓕ	119 ⓣ ⓕ	149 ⓣ ⓕ
30 ⓣ ⓕ	60 ⓣ ⓕ	90 ⓣ ⓕ	120 ⓣ ⓕ	150 ⓣ ⓕ

Sample computer sheet, reproduced by kind permission of the Royal College of General Practitioners.

MCQ PRACTICE EXAM

Time allowed 2 hours.

Gallstones

1   have a prevalence of over 50% in subjects over 65 years of age
2   typically occur in subjects taking a diet with a high fibre content
3   are symptomless in the majority
4   the majority are radio-opaque
5   typically respond poorly to medical therapy

Crohn's disease

6   the incidence of Crohn's disease is decreasing in the United Kingdom
7   large bowel involvement is less common in the elderly
8   about 70% of cases eventually require surgery
9   erythema nodosum is a characteristic feature
10   pericholangitis is an associated feature

Causes of pruritus ani include

11   poor anal hygiene
12   eczema
13   diabetes
14   Hodgkin's disease
15   pediculosis

The following diseases are notifiable in England and Wales:

16   whooping cough
17   tuberculosis
18   malaria
19   rubella
20   acute meningitis

Results in clinical papers

21 small differences in results can be amplified by logarithmic scales
22 the median is the average value
23 the mode is equal to the mean
24 the range is the distribution, from the highest to the lowest value
25 the standard deviation expresses the numbers around the mean for a particular value

Schneider's first-rank symptoms of schizophrenia include

26 thought insertion
27 thought broadcasting
28 flattening of affect
29 poverty of speech
30 voices discussing the patient's thoughts or behaviour

In bulimia nervosa

31 cognitive behavioural therapy has been shown to be effective
32 group therapy has been shown to be ineffective
33 the prognosis is worse than for anorexia nervosa
34 vomiting is a recognised accompaniment

Acute confusional states are more likely when the following are present:

35 hypothyroidism
36 bronchopneumonia
37 an unstimulating environment
38 treatment with benzodiazepines
39 increasing age

The following factors are associated with physical abuse of a child (non-accidental injury):

40 age under two years
41 obstetric complications
42 poor mothering ability noted in the postnatal ward
43 criminality in the parents
44 illegitimacy

In polymyalgia rheumatica

45   men are more often affected than women
46   the presence of fever rules out the diagnosis
47   the serum alkaline phosphatase is raised in the majority
48   ESR is normal in 5% of subjects
49   treatment should be continued for a minimum of 2 years

Acute pericarditis

50   is most commonly the result of myocardial infarction
51   causes pain which is worse when sitting up
52   characteristically causes ECG changes
53   has been shown to develop within a few hours of myocardial infarction

Recurrent aphthous ulceration of the mouth

54   has been shown to have an autoimmune basis in some patients
55   has no hereditary basis
56   may remit during pregnancy
57   is commonly associated with food intolerance
58   is commonly precipitated or aggravated by smoking

Recognised causes of urinary incontinence include

59   previous radiotherapy
60   multiple sclerosis
61   Parkinson's disease
62   diabetic neuropathy
63   faecal impaction

Recognised causes of macrocytosis include

64   alcoholism
65   chronic renal failure
66   hypothyroidism
67   aplastic anaemia
68   cytotoxic drug therapy

In patients with obstructive sleep apnoea syndrome, there is an increased incidence of the following:

69   systemic hypertension
70   pulmonary hypertension
71   daytime somnolence
72   polycythaemia
73   depression

A tremor of the outstretched hands

74   typically responds to propranolol
75   is often familial and benign
76   may be worsened by anxiety
77   is improved by primidone

The following are true of the acquired immunodeficiency syndrome (AIDS):

78   it is a notifiable disease
79   *Pneumocystis carinii* pneumonia has a characteristic X-ray appearance
80   diarrhoea due to cryptosporidium responds to metronidazole
81   it has been shown to cause presenile dementia
82   it cannot be diagnosed without a positive serological test

In the assessment of proteinuria discovered unexpectedly at routine examination

83   proteinuria may persist for years without progressive renal impairment
84   orthostatic proteinuria is always benign
85   it may be secondary to analgesic abuse
86   it is usually secondary to a lower urinary tract infection

Recognised manifestations of diabetes mellitus in children include

87   growth retardation
88   precocious puberty
89   weight loss
90   increased psychiatric morbidity
91   microvascular disease

In urinary tract infection in children

92 5% of school girls have asymptomatic bacteriuria
93 the incidence in boys and girls is equal in the first year of life
94 vesicoureteric reflux (VUR) is present in 70% of cases when first seen
95 patients with VUR when first seen nearly always have established renal scarring
96 no structural abnormality can be demonstrated in half the cases

The following are typical of developmental delay:

97 not responding to name at 1 year
98 no distinct word at 15 months
99 not walking at 20 months
100 casting of objects at 14 months
101 not sitting alone at 8 months

Atopic eczema in the infant characteristically affects the

102 cheeks
103 antecubital fossae
104 folds of the neck
105 groin
106 popliteal fossae

Lichen planus

107 causes intense itching
108 typically begins in childhood
109 produces depigmented lesions in coloured subjects
110 has a natural tendency to spontaneous remission
111 should not be treated with topical corticosteroids

Recognised causes of generalised pruritus include

112 pregnancy
113 hyperthyroidism
114 iron overload
115 drug abuse
116 aplastic anaemia

The following drugs have been shown to cause gynaecomastia:

117 cyproterone acetate
118 tamoxifen
119 cyclophosphamide
120 imipramine
121 danazol

The following side effects have been shown to occur with the use of trimethoprim:

122 megaloblastic anaemia
123 Stevens-Johnson syndrome
124 fever
125 diarrhoea
126 headaches

The dose of warfarin may need to be reduced if any of the following drugs are given in addition:

127 cimetidine
128 erythromycin
129 sulphinpyrazone
130 cholestyramine
131 rifampicin

Teratogenicity

132 sodium valproate has been shown to be associated with an increased risk of spina bifida
133 phenytoin is associated with congenital heart disease
134 carbamazepine is associated with bone marrow depression
135 lithium carbonate is associated with congenital heart disease
136 heparin causes c.n.s. defects

The following drugs have been shown to alter the quantity of maternal milk secretion:

137 ethanol
138 metoclopramide
139 lithium
140 aspirin
141 bromocriptine

The menopause

142 cigarette smoking is associated with a later menopause
143 hot flushes usually present before the psychological symptoms of the menopause
144 hot flushes are more likely to occur during menstruation
145 myocardial infarction is an absolute contra-indication to hormone replacement treatment

Vaginal discharge

146 oral contraception may decrease vaginal secretions
147 *Trichomonas vaginalis* is associated with a white discharge
148 *Streptococcus faecalis* is a common cause of acute salpingo-oophoritis

Hyperemesis gravidarum

149 is associated with multiple pregnancy
150 causes renal damage
151 occurs most commonly in primigravida
152 is associated with fetal abnormality

Asymptomatic bacteriuria in pregnancy

153 is found in approximately 20% of pregnant women
154 is associated with an increased rate of premature delivery
155 is associated with anaemia
156 is associated with an increased rate of foetal abnormalities
157 is associated with decreased mean birth weight

Diabetes in pregnancy is associated with the following:

158 pre-eclamptic toxaemia
159 cardiac malformations in the foetus
160 an increased incidence of post-partum haemorrhage
161 slowing of progression of maternal retinopathy

Carpal tunnel syndrome

162 may present with pain in the forearm
163 is associated with fasciculation of the small muscles of the hand
164 is exacerbated by coughing and sneezing
165 is typically bilateral

The following are recognised features of rheumatoid arthritis (RA):

166 exacerbation during pregnancy
167 scleritis
168 dry mouth
169 sacroiliitis
170 leg ulceration

The period of incubation is less than seven days for

171 diphtheria
172 mumps
173 rubella
174 scarlet fever
175 malaria

Hearing problems in the elderly

176 presbycousis is an age related phenomenon
177 presbycousis is rarely associated with abnormal loudness perception
178 tinnitus has a prevalence of 10% in the sixth decade
179 tinnitus is always associated with hearing loss
180 two hearing aids are better than one

Diabetes in the elderly

181 diagnosis in the 60s or 70s has not been shown to affect life expectancy
182 pruritus vulvae is a recognised presentation
183 retinopathy is typically found in maturity onset diabetics
184 is associated with increased cataract formation

Glaucoma

185 the incidence is about 1% of those over 65
186 loss of vision may occur over a few days
187 coloured halos may apear around lights
188 the pupil may be small and react sluggishly to light
189 may be precipitated by tricyclic antidepressants

When removing patients from your list

190 the practice manager should inform the FHSA
191 a reason should be given
192 the patient is removed as soon as he/she joins another practice or 14 days later, whichever is the sooner
193 patients cannot be removed if they are receiving treatment at intervals of less than a week

Rules regarding doctors availability state

194 full time principles will normally be available for 46 weeks in any period of 12 months
195 full time principles should be available for not less than 26 hours in each week on 5 days in each week
196 GPs involved in the improvement of quality of care may be available on only 4 days per week
197 hours of availability may include time spent on home visits

The practice leaflet must contain

198 the full names of the doctors
199 age of doctors
200 how to obtain an urgent and non-urgent appointment
201 whether minor surgery is provided
202 how patients can make complaints about the practice

The medical audit advisory group

203 exists to encourage GPs to undertake audit in their practice
204 has a legal duty to investigate complaints against GPs
205 exists to inform the FHSA which practices have performed satisfactory audits
206 must be facilitated by the FHSA
207 may develop a database of audits which can be used by individual practices

Claims for treating patients not on your list

208 a temporary resident form (FP19) should not be completed if a visiting patient only requests contraception
209 if you treat a patient who you do not wish to take on your list you should complete an emergency treatment form (FP32)
210 if you are called to attend a patient who is visiting from Romania you will not be paid via the FHSA

The health and safety at work act (1974) legislation states

211 the provision and maintenance of a working environment should be safe and provide adequate facilities
212 the legislation also covers the health and safety of the patients using the premises
213 a written statement of policy with respect to health and safety should be provided by anyone who employs staff
214 under the act an employer may not charge an employee for any protective clothing they require for work

Gastric carcinoma

215 incidence in the UK is declining
216 is associated with previous surgery to the stomach
217 most tumours are palpable on first presentation
218 is associated with hyperacidity
219 lymph node spread is rare

Bronchial carcinoma

220 causes 2000 deaths per year in England
221 the majority of primary tumours are caused by adenocarcinomas
222 may present with dementia
223 involvement of the sympathetic chain may cause a Horner's syndrome

Epidemiology of ischaemic heart disease (IHD)

224 over 70% of deaths certified as IHD have not been investigated, occur
     at home and are certified without post-mortem
225 death rates are high in northern European and English speaking
     countries and low in southern European countries
226 there is a raised incidence of IHD in hard water areas
227 IHD is the cause of 10% of deaths in most western countries

**The following factors in a suicidal attempt suggest that the attempt was a
serious one:**

228 extensive premeditation (more than 3 hours)
229 telling others of the intention before the attempt
230 leaving a suicide note
231 admitting suicidal intent
232 making a will beforehand

Agoraphobic patients

233 are typically female
234 often have a fear of fainting
235 benefit from aversion therapy
236 the majority have marital problems
237 may report depersonalisation

Munchausen's syndrome is characterised by

238 female sex
239 delusions of illness
240 obsessional personality
241 folie a deux
242 recovery after surgical intervention

Recognised associations of hypothyroidism include

243 pericardial effusion
244 erythema ab igne
245 menorrhagia
246 cerebellar ataxia
247 normochromic anaemia

The following are correct statements concerning palpitations:

248 in the majority of patients palpitations are not associated with primary heart disease
249 paroxysmal tachycardias seldom occur on a daily basis
250 the usual explanation of 'dropped beats' is ectopic activity
251 ectopic beats are commoner when the heart rate is relatively slow

In acute gout

252 fever may occur
253 the first attack is characteristically monarticular
254 the plasma urate is always raised
255 the synovial fluid may be purulent
256 the drug of choice is indomethacin

In the treatment of acute hepatitis due to hepatitis A virus

257 the patient should be nursed in isolation for 10 days after the appearance of jaundice
258 strict bed-rest during this period is advisable
259 drugs should be avoided unless absolutely necessary
260 the period of convalescence should be approximately twice the symptomatic period

In long-term domiciliary oxygen therapy for obstructive airways disease with oedema

261 the oxygen must be given for at least 15 hours per day if survival is to improve

262 no further improvement in survival is gained by prolonging therapy for more than 6 months

263 if oxygen concentrator is used, the emergent gas contains at least 90% of oxygen

264 the most efficient mode of delivery with an oxygen concentrator is via nasal cannulae

Characteristic findings in normal pressure hydrocephalus include

265 mental deterioration

266 onset before puberty

267 incontinence

268 papilloedema

269 enlargement of the ventricles

Published guidelines for management of asthma suggest

270 patients who need to inhale a bronchodilator more than once daily require regular inhaled anti-inflammatory drugs

271 a short course of steroids is indicated if peak expiratory flow falls below 60% of patients best result

272 patients should be encouraged to start oral steroids on their own initiative

273 patients on maintenance oral steroids should have their inhaled steroid treatment stopped

274 in an acute attack oxygen therapy should be used at 28% concentration

Recognised findings in babies affected by the fetal alcohol syndrome include

275 microcephaly

276 high birth weight

277 abnormal palmar creases

278 cardiac septal defects

279 deformities of the fingers

In the examination of the newborn

280 the absence of the Moro reflex is not of serious significance
281 a congenital dermal sinus may cause meningitis
282 three vessels in the cord may indicate renal abnormality
283 umbilical hernias are an indication for surgery
284 a high pitched cry may be a sign of cerebral irritability

Rosacea

285 is commoner in men than in women
286 typically improves on exposure to sunshine
287 will usually improve spontaneously within 6-10 weeks
288 responds to treatment with tetracycline
289 responds to treatment with topical corticosteroids

Biguanides

290 are contra-indicated in the obese diabetic
291 have been shown to interact with cimetidine
292 in overdose cause hypoglycaemia in normal subjects
293 if given to patients with reduced renal function increase the risk of lactic acidosis
294 are associated with a metallic taste if given with alcohol

Nitrate tolerance

295 tolerance to the adverse effects indicates tolerance to the therapeutic effects
296 typically takes at least one month to develop
297 topical nitrates have been shown not to produce tolerance
298 isosorbide mononitrate has been shown to produce less tolerance than isosorbide dinitrate
299 once developed is permanent

Absorption of the following drugs has been shown to be increased if they are given on an empty stomach:

300 digoxin
301 allopurinol
302 co-trimoxazole
303 theophylline
304 penicillins

Genital herpes

305 usually has an incubation period of 4-5 days
306 characteristically causes a mild first attack, followed by recurrences of increasing severity
307 can most accurately be confirmed by cell culture
308 is resistant to all anti-viral agents

Pre-menstrual tension

309 PMT is significantly more common in women with a high degree of neuroticism
310 PMT is exacerbated by diabetes
311 vitamin B6 is thought to be of benefit by helping dopamine production
312 a diet including celery, cucumber, nuts and fried foods may help alleviate symptoms
313 epidemiological studies show that about 60% of women experience PMT at some time

A patient with a haemoglobin level of 9.2 g/dl at 34 weeks gestation

314 should have a bone marrow test performed
315 should be given an iron infusion
316 should have a blood transfusion
317 is likely to have iron deficiency anaemia

Antimicrobial treatment is advisable for

318 *Salmonella* gastroenteritis
319 *Shigella sonnei* infection
320 typhoid fever
321 giardiasis
322 *Yersinia* infections if severe

Transient ischaemic attacks (TIA)

323 full recovery occurs within 12 hours
324 TIAs originating in the vertebra-basilar region have a worse prognosis
325 aspirin is more effective at preventing TIAs in males
326 both carotid and vertebra-basilar TIAs may cause speech problems
327 carotid endarterectomy should be considered if carotid stenosis is present

Nitrazepam in the elderly has been shown to cause the following:

328 nightmares
329 hypothermia
330 osteomalacia
331 ataxia

Senile cataracts

332 always develop gradually
333 referral is not required until the cataract has reached an advanced stage
334 when advanced prevent perception of light and dark
335 may present with diplopia

Squint

336 children do not grow out of a true squint
337 treatment is rarely successful after the age of 6
338 the main aim of treatment is to restore binocular vision
339 may be secondary to retinoblastoma
340 may be suspected in a child who persistently tilts his head

New patient registration consultations

341   must be offered to all patients over 5 years of age
342   chest and heart must be examined
343   a fee may only be claimed if the consultation is performed within
      6 weeks of registering

**Doctors may accept fees from NHS patients under the following
circumstances:**

344   there is no evidence the patient is on the list
345   prescribing anti-malarial pills for travel abroad
346   road traffic accidents
347   completing a disability living allowance application form

Cervical cytology target

348   the women included in the target are those between 20 and 65
349   the higher target means that 80% of the women must have had a smear
      under general medical services
350   women who have had a recent smear with a previous GP are not
      counted towards payment by your practice
351   the FHSA require a list of patients who have had a complete
      hysterectomy
352   women who have never been sexually active are excluded from the
      target

Access to health records

353   patients are entitled to see all their medical records
354   no charge may be made to the patient
355   access may be denied, if in the opinion of the holder, it would cause
      harm to the health of the patient
356   corrections may be made to the notes if requested by the patient

Employment rules state

357   businesses employing more than 20 employees must take on a quota of 3% registered disabled persons

358   employers must not expect the same standard of work from disabled people

359   an employee does not require a minimum period of notice to leave if employed for less than 1 year

360   employers are required by law to insure against liabilities to staff sustained during their employment

THE MODIFIED ESSAY QUESTION PAPER

INTRODUCTION

The MEQ is a form of assessment pioneered by the College and it is in this paper that candidates score lowest. If the MCQ is regarded as testing knowledge then the MEQ looks instead at problem-solving skills and behaviour and favours the candidate who thinks widely. It assesses the candidate's ability to identify the nature of a presented problem and to propose a range of solutions. To some extent it also seeks to identify and evaluate the candidate's attitude to the situations described.

The MEQ has, like the rest of the exam, been modified over the years. At the present time it is presented as a series of ten situations that might be encountered in a typical day in general practice. These situations are mostly independent, although there may be some connection between them. The main areas covered are:

1. Clinical diagnosis and management. This includes information gathering, hypothesis formation, preparation of management plans and therapy with anticipation of possible future problems.
2. Preventive medicine including protocol development and assessment.
3. 'Problem' and 'difficult' patients.
4. Psychological and social problems affecting individuals and families.
5. The consultation process.
6. Practice organisation including Primary Health Care Team.
7. Relationships with colleagues and others.
8. Recognition of doctor's own feelings.
9. Appreciation of ethical and medico-legal problems.

Each situation is described in a few lines at the top of a separate page, the remainder of the page and its reverse are available for your answer. The answer should be in expanded note form, to allow the maximum amount of information to be written down in the allowed time. However, your writing should be legible and use of arbitrary abbreviations avoided.

Good exam technique requires an appreciation of the relationship between the marks gained and the length of time spent answering the questions. Each question carries equal marks and it is therefore very important to answer **each** question as fully as possible. This requires strict time management.

The total time allocation for the paper is only 2 hours i.e. 12 minutes per question.

After the exam, the MEQ paper is separated into the individual questions each of which is forwarded to a different examiner for marking. Since each examiner is only marking one question, it is important to answer each question fully even if it means repeating what you have stated in the previous answer.

The marking schedule for each question is developed by pooling the answers of a group of examiners who have answered the question themselves. This produces a range of possible answers which are then ranked by 'appropriateness'. Candidates' grades are decided by comparing their answers against those of the combined examiners.

The following are typical questions:

- Outline your management.
- What use would you make of this consultation?
- What issues would you discuss with this patient?
- What problems does this present?
- Summarise the problems that you will need to address.
- How would you decide what to do?
- How would you respond?
- What issues does this presentation present?
- What responses are possible and what might be their consequences?
- What are the possible implications of this change?
- What would be your criteria for this patient's effective care?
- What is your role in further care?
- Speculate on the issues and problems which may concern the patient in the future.

Answering this type of question well is not easy! Having a structured approach is essential.

1. Read the initial MEQ instructions – they may be different to what you expect!
2. Read the scenario carefully, for nearly every word has some significance.

3. Think in broad terms about the whole of the case, not just about the superficial symptom or diagnosis described.
4. Think what areas the question is exploring. This helps you to see into the examiner's mind when he was setting the question. A question superficially about acne may be an ethical dilemma rather than a clinical challenge!
5. Imagine how you yourself would deal with such a problem in your day-to-day care.
6. Remember to limit yourself to twelve minutes per question.

It is useful to have a mental framework to help you structure your answers and this will ensure that you are thinking broadly and producing a range of options.

The value of such a framework is to provide a clear thought pathway when you feel anxious and confused. All or part of each framework may be used singly or in combination.

Examples of frameworks are as follows:

A problem solving approach
A – Assessment. Consider all problem areas.
P – Plan. Decide what needs to be done.
I – Implementation. Decide who does what, when and where. Consider delegation.
E – Evaluation.

A model for the consultation
1. **Explore** the patient's knowledge, ideas, concerns, expectations.
2. **Explain** their symptoms and signs.
3. **Consider** the treatment options.
4. **Advise** the patient on options.
5. **Consider** the patient's preference.
6. **Involve** the patient in the management plan.

Aspects of the consultation
Management of presenting problems
Management of continuing problems
Modification of help-seeking behaviour
Opportunistic health promotion

Consider the implications for the following:
Patient
Doctor
Practice
Primary Health Care Team
Hospital
Family and Carers

Management options
R – Reassure
A – Advise
P – Prescribe. To give script or not.
R – Refer. To whom?
I   – Investigate
O – Observe and follow up

Giving bad news
A – Anxiety: try to elicit patient's anxieties.
K – Knowledge: try to elicit patient's knowledge.
E – Explanation: diagnosis in simple terms, prognosis, treatment and follow up.
S – Sympathy and support.

Dealing with anger
A – Avoid confrontation
F – Facilitate discussion
V – Ventilate feelings
E – Explore reasons
R – Refer/investigate

Problem areas
Physical
Psychological
Social   e.g. Finance
            Housing
            Work
            Family
            Leisure
            Sex

Consider an example:
Mrs Smith aged 54 enquires about hormone replacement therapy because she has heard that it helps prevent future osteoporosis. What factors would you like to take into account in considering your reply.

This question involves an appreciation of the following areas:
- Clinical knowledge
- Prevention
- Consultation process including health beliefs
- Patient autonomy
- Choice.

You could use the framework **A model for the consultation,** described earlier, this would ensure that all the necessary areas are included. Your final answer should include:
- Discussion of expectations of treatment, based on health beliefs.
- Enquire about any possible false beliefs.
- Enquire into present health and past medical history, with specific reference to HRT benefits and side effects.
- Include family history and lifestyle factors.
- Exploration of what prompted the attendance and 'why now'.
- Explanation of risk/side effect versus benefit ratio.
- Respect of patient's wishes and choice.
- Explanation of 'non HRT factors' influencing osteoporosis.

In order to gain maximum marks each topic needs to be expanded with appropriate facts. Marking is based on a conceptual marking system in which the examiner grades various concepts rather than a mere factual 'tick list'. For a good pass answer the candidate would need to be aware of at least half the issues, and to address most of them reasonably well. For a fail, fewer than half the issues would be noted, and dealt with superficially. The standard of pass/fail (the cutting edge) is decided by the individual examiner, following a discussion with his fellow marking colleagues at the annual examiners' meeting. Research has shown that there is good correlation among examiners in ranking candidates.

INSTRUCTIONS FOR THE PRACTICE MEQ PAPERS

Two practice MEQ papers are presented on the following pages.

Your answers should be brief and may take the form of lists rather than lengthy descriptions.

The answers and marking schedules for these MEQs are to be found at the end of this book, but do not turn to these pages until you have written your own answers in the space provided.

1. There are ten questions in the MEQ paper. Total time allowed is 2 hours.

2. Answers should be brief, legible and concise.

3. Answers should be written in the space provided. If more room is required use additional paper.

4. You are advised not to alter your answers after completing the whole MEQ and not to look through the pages before you start. This may distort your natural assessment of the case and cause you to lose marks.

5. Each page of the MEQ is marked independently. You should therefore answer each question fully even if this answer involves repetition of part of an earlier answer.

6. As a rough guide it is indicated when you are approximately halfway through this paper.

MEQ PRACTICE PAPER 1

Write your answers in the space provided.
Time allowed: 2 hours.

1. You are a partner in a five doctor group practice, working from a purpose
   built Health Centre. The appointment system allows an average of seven
   and a half minutes per consultation.

   Your first patient, Mrs Smith, is new to the practice. What are the main
   points you would like to discuss with her at this consultation?

Consultation ; Time Mx ; Delegation

① welcome her to practice.   Has she a practice leaflet
                                    ? delegate
② ?Has she had new reg. check   ? do it self

③ Is there a presenting complaint - deal with this

④ Take PMH, PSH - Social history - include smoking, etoH
exercise + diet (for HP) . Obstetric hx
DH - Allergies ; FH   × BP
Imms? : give tetanus   Ht, wt^ ∘ ask for urinalysis
      Last smear

⑤ Allow her to discuss problems ; concerns ; any Qu's

⑥ ~~other~~ Social - why has she joined
                    - how is she moving in etc

⑦ with leaflet - discuss practical / workings of surgeries
    - visits ; repeat Rx ; other services
    - ? delegate to someone else

2. Mrs Brown brings in her eight and a half year old son Tom and tells you that he is due to go on a school holiday in four weeks time, but she is worried because he is still wetting the bed most nights. How can you help?

Short term / long term

Problem solving approach. Physical, psych., Social

Assess — empathise + allow her to express ideas, concerns + expectations

① Take history — 1° or 2° ; ? during day
— any other Sx ; organic cause
— psychological or emotional problems — school + sibs
— FH ; birth Hx ; position in family
— recent life events

② Examine — unlikely find any abn

③ Ix — take MSU ; urinalysis

④ Mx — depends on cause. Include Tom in decisions
— but if 1° — reassure mother
— explain normals
— can be $\bar{n}$, but behavioural

Rx can help / cure

what has been tried so far — ↓ fluids
— ? lifting
— ? star chart
— pad / bell

? deal by self ? refer to community paediatrician
child psych ; HV

Any other developmental abn

Reassure that can cope with holiday by
supplying short term Rx = tricyclics — imipramine
or desmopressin

? Involve school / teachers

Long term Rx — pad + bell
— ? family therapy

3. Stan Bridge is a 58 year old labourer who has just been diagnosed as having angina. He has been started on atenolol and is awaiting a consultant outpatient appointment. His angina initially seemed to be well controlled but now he complains of chest pain on exertion. Why might Stan's angina not be improving?

Pt factors; Doctor factors; Drugs. Physical; ψ; social.

Reassure r develop rapport Allow him to express ideas, concerns

Take history - enquire as to ① Is he taking tabs?
                                        compliance

② - right dose   - s/e
Has he ↑ activity after starting Rx ∴ → ↑ Sx
Is he worried it might something else ? Psychological aspects
Does he understand disease   -is he depressed?

③ financial factors - can he afford Rx   anxious
                                      Rejecting Δ
Doctor
    ? right diagnosis
    ? right Rx - may need to change it. needs

GTN
    ↑ anxiety not noted
    ? Unstable angina
    ? MI - ⇒ urgent referral
Is he taking other general advice
  ? o/w wife - ? confidentiality
d/w Consultant   ? earlier / urgent
        - arrange ECG

4. Susan, a sixteen year old schoolgirl, comes in crying accompanied by her mother. Her mother demands that Susan goes on the oral contraceptive pill. Outline the different approaches available to you for this consultation.

Family dynamics ; consultation skills ; confidentiality & ethics

Allow silence & for agendas to emerge. Why now? what has happened? eg.

Would Susan prefer to be seen alone?

① See Susan _ what's happened?
              -? risk of pregnancy ?having sex
              - does she want to go on pill?
              - history / risk factors / CI / SE
              - is she mature enough to understand
              - using other methods of contraception
              - information is confidential   - Emergency

- may antagonise mother
                  - smears - inform

② Discuss with jointly?
          - what the problems are
          - problems in family   - mother + daughter
                      - family

Allow both to express concerns
Pt autonomy - she has right to choose

F.U   - see Susan alone & develop trust

?involve PHCT

5. Mr Partridge, a 62 year old railwayman, is concerned that he is having to spend increasing amounts of time looking after his wife, who has just had a dense hemiplegic stroke. He asks your advice on whether he should retire or not. How do you respond to this?

Marital relationships? Coping at home? Hidden agendas?

- Empathise - difficult looking after disabled relative

Why now?

Problems for Mr. Partridge — allow him to express worries

① can't cope — ↑ physical problems of own ? "call for help"
  - psychological problems - depressed /anxi:
  - emotional - difficult seeing wife like this

② Can he cope financially — pension
  - DLA
  - benefits
  - ! hidden agendas ? guilt

Loss of independence — social contact
  - ! enjoys job
  - may tend to resentment

Can he get other family to help ? other services HV, SS; DN

Wife — ↑ demanding :↑ unable to cope
  ? respite care :DN

Doctor — give him the facts — help out as you can
He must make an informed decision
  - Rx underlying problems
  - involves helpers PHCT, SS, voluntary agencies
  - appreciate stress of carers ↑now & his feeling are n

YOU ARE NOW APPROXIMATELY HALF WAY THROUGH THIS PAPER
  - help him to consider pros & cons of retirement
  in psychological, financial & social terms
  ? he may already have made up his mind to retire &
  just want reinforcement
  - what do wife, friends, relatives & employer think
  - arrange f/u

51

6. Your next patient, Marjorie Holme, is a 53 year old teacher and she produces a written sheet of paper from her handbag and says that she requires
   a) your opinion of a 'mole' on her back
   b) some cream for her eczema
   c) a repeat script for her hormone replacement therapy
   d) some antibiotics for her husband's 'bad chest' —ethical dilemma

   What issues are raised by this form of presentation? feelings in doctor

Educated pt - ? changing role ? demanding. Consultation model.
written requests   Multiple Px - time Mx
   Allow silence - if feel resentment/anger —allow it to subside
① List writer -may engender feeling in doctor

Does she always do this ?
   ? Is she a heartsink or demanding pt

May not be able to deal with all issues in
one consultation : what are most important
- Don't want to rush her - but will have to
return . Time for her, self & other pt's

Each may be extended problem in itself.

Also, are she & husband very busy - & is that
why they 'save up' & present in this way
? disorganised home life
? difficulty coping
empathise with her , but be firm & ask he
to return.
pt's autonomy & has right to choose agenda
   ? hidden agendas

7. Mr Jones, aged 56, attends for a 'well man' health check and on urinalysis is found to have 2% glycosuria, but no ketones. His weight is 140 kilograms and he smokes 25 cigarettes per day. Outline your management plan at this stage.

Consultation; Breaking bad news ; Health advice ; F.u

will have developed rapport and know how much info he can handle at one go

would want to confirm Δ of diabetes
— B.G - now
& arrange
— inform pt of your suspicions   Fasting B.G + HbA1c
— reassure him   — explain natural hx /S/signs   Lipids
                                                                          u+E's

Take a history   have suspicions of disease →why ho
        — did he
attended check
        — FH   — any experience of disease.
        — diet
Examine — general . Neuro ; eyes ;
Ix- — q/a Baseline ? end organ damage
Mx — Inform . Involve pt in decisions . Practice
                                                    (protocol)
        — Can be mild disease — modify diet &
                                            — medical Mx
weight — may control
        — refer to diabetic nurse & consultant
                — dietician
                — given written material /leaflets.
        Allow him to express his ideas & concerns
                                            — ask Qu's
        What he thinks is going to happen
        Give advice re other risk factors — exercise ; smoking
        Arrange f.u   Involve family
        Also — & occupational — problems
                                — ? driving — notify DVLA   **53**
                                            & car insurance

8. Mrs Morton comes in alone, saying that she is worried about her husband Michael who is drinking 8 pints of beer each night. What issues does this presentation present?

2nd hand info. Why now? ? Ethics + confidential
Cry for help

Why now?
Why has she come alone — not with husband.
what has been going on? — is he your pt
? true facts ? hidden agenda

Can empathise, and say you are unable to do anything without her husband there!

offer support & advice †

what are problems for him — financial ; physical
— social
—why is he drinking —work; driving
—recent or long term — legal
— violent; emotional

for her? — violence ; financial
— physical worries about him

family
Give advice — he can attend by self; with
her or you will tackle at next appt
— information re: addiction clinic
AA

offer F.U.
? Difficult to get husband to co-operate
Hidden agenda — wife's own problems
? breach of confidentiality

54

9. Your next patient is Linda Brown, a 38 year old sewing machinist who bursts into tears as soon as she sits down. She says that she cannot cope with life any longer. What are your aims for this consultation?

Consultation technique?

Allow silence for her to express her concerns /worries /anxieties . Establish rapport
Empathise and allow her to elaborate . Develop trust

(1) what is going on now? ─ physical, social
        ─ how long? ─ Psychological
        ─ initiated by?
                                            4x × FX

(2) MSE ─ is she depressed; suicidal
        ─ what has she tried

(3) Mx ─ what support network does she have
                            ─ coping strategies
        ─ what can you do for her ─ joint
arrangement
        ─ time constraints ─ make another appt +

discuss more fully with double appt
        ∴ short term anxiolytic
        ─ antidepressive
─ refer CPN /SW
─ refer +
─ Reassure ; F.U ; "always available"
    Allow time to recover ─ "house-keeping"

10. Two days later, you are telephoned by the local hospital to say that Linda Brown has taken a fatal overdose of paracetamol. You feel very upset that despite all your care and support Linda Brown has killed herself. What strategies are available to you in helping you to deal with these emotions?

Feeling in self - anger, guilt ; sadness ; fear
-coping mechanism

Acknowledge feelings in self
    —take time out to think it over
    —? look through notes
    —d/w doctors at hospital what happened
    — make contact with family — they may
blame you —   allow them to express. Show you
—so now ; —has right to take life
    —pt autonomy —anger— 'could have helped
d/w other partners   —feelings in self
            —seek reassurance
            — 'did all you could'
    ?guilt — should have recognised risk

d/w spouse/friends   —   support ? see women
seek more professional help —but doctors wary
                    of this
May affect you in future consultations
? consider post-poning oncall or major decision
Be aware of risk of _____

MEQ PRACTICE PAPER 2

Write your answers in the space provided.
Time allowed: 2 hours.

1. You are a partner in a three doctor inner city practice. Morning surgery begins with Nancy Colt, a 19 year old single parent who brings her 18 month old son Lee and complains that he will not sleep at night. One of her friends lent her some 'sleeping medicine' which she had given to Lee with good effect. She asks you to prescribe some for Lee. Outline your management.

[Handwritten notes:]

being single parent - ? coping ? social situation ? extended family
- ethical ; demanding. feelings in pt / in doctor
Consultation technique

Be empathetic & develop rapport Listen to her concerns
& ideas. Be understanding - develop trust Allow silences
why now?
① Take history - Lee - PM - other problems - difficult child
- physical problems
- worries -
- does he seem well
- checks limms 4TJ ?h/o abuse/neglect

Mother - ? psychology / emotional & social disorder
- 'end of letter'
- hidden agenda ? coping
- support network / family ? ss involved
- ? HIV

Mx amen problem - what is the pattern
what has been tried - regular routine
behavioural ↓ noise
Advise on , techniques : explain N
Pt education Involve Nancy
May need medication short-term - both for mother
& baby - but emphasise - discuss risks & s/e
- Involve HV refer to amen ? referral
- offer support & F.U

2. Mr Joseph, a 72 year old retired tailor, requests a transfer onto your list from that of a neighbouring doctor. He has not recently changed address. What are the possible reasons for such a request?

Pt factors ; family ; Doctor factors ; Practice /organisation
/staff

→ why now?

Pt ⌐ Underlying dissatisfaction — searching different opinion
?recent change in doctor ? difficult pt -argument
-technique /methods / organisation

would like change
feels it is closer /easier access /more services
Heard about it from family /friends
Ex family on your list .

Doctor
Different type of practice
? better rapport /friends
hidden agenda
-manipulate
Services
Try out new doctors ? more amenable new doctor
? false expectation- quicker Rx
On-going medical problem - different approach
? wrong Δ c̄ other

Staff ⌐ friends.
Practice ⌐ change in the practice - ? moved e: cơ dơ hulls
Difficult getting appts
Change in access.

Realise ease of change now
? feelings ur doctor - ? ↑ income as ↑ work
Selection on positive vs. negative grounds

58

3. Your next patient, Mavis Hawke, a 58 year old office cleaner, comes for the result of her recent chest X-ray. For the last six months she has had a cough and more recently haemoptysis. The report shows a right hilar mass and a shadow in the right upper zone, consistent with a bronchial carcinoma. How would you proceed with this consultation?

Consultation technique ; Breaking Bad news.
- Rapport
welcome ; Enable her to express her ideas, concerns
+ expectations - She may have idea - of what is wrong
present state . Appropriate setting - quiet & uninterrupted
also, than pt aware of bad news
Judge as to how much she will take in &
understand and in what language.
? Is she accompanied by family
Once established trust & rapport
Inform her of CXR results - the most likely
diagnosis.
    Allow her some time to express anxieties
                                    - beware - denial, disbelief, anger
Difficult for her to accept & take in anything
- shock, worry for self ; family   Pace consultation
    - give her information regarding disease. What does she know?
    - what to do next   - further consultation with
specialist ; further Ix ; follow-up Rx   Δ
            ? cure / palliative   prognosis
In-volve family   Rx
F.U are sympathy/support /counselling emotional / Ψ.   F.U
feeling in doctor - difficult to break news
            - allow time to get over consultation
Consider Mx present Sx eg cough
Review any medication

4. **Carl Gatsby, a twenty year old student, asks for advice about his forthcoming six month trip to South East Asia. He asks 'What jabs and things do I need, Doctor?'. What sources of information are available to enable you to advise this patient fully?**

Imms² ; health style advice ; risk groups
Pt centred ; Doctor centred

<u>Assess</u>

When is he going?
Where is he going? to do what
Is he generally well? Any chronic conditions
UTD ⃝ imms? which ones will he need?
Malaria - tabs + general measures
Advice STD ; AIDS -
Eating & drinking - & on
Advice - danger areas ; insurance
Diseases endemic to area
Social - have a good time

<u>Information</u>

Medical press - Pulse , Doctor , MIM's charts
- other journals BNF
London School of Tropical diseases - DHSS leaflet SA40
Phone-lines - advice to travellers
DoH guidelines
Embassies ; Prestel or Travel companies

Be aware <u>variety of</u> information eg Thomas Cook

5. Mrs Richards enters, very upset. She says her mother-in-law aged 82 years, who lives with her, is 'saying things' and talking to herself. Mrs Richards feels that she cannot cope any longer and would like her mother-in-law to be admitted to hospital permanently. How would you respond?

Relatives request = out pt? Pt autonomy? Ethics
Why now? Problem solving

① Sympathise + emphathise. Allow her to express ideas, concerns , what she should think happen

② why now? How long has she been coping at home? Any help? SS? Family? End of tether? ? Calling card — problems social, + emotional on Mrs R.
acute problem

③ Take hx r/ Mother in law — how long?
— other Sx?
medical social — ? organic cause
& psychological — ? psychological / emotional cause
— ? dementia

will need to arrange time to visit & assess
— will this be possible. any new
? arrange DV c consultant . medical
— ask DN; H.V of elderly ; SS
— will she allow referral referral is appropriate
— Examine on home visit

④ Affect on Mrs. R & rest of family
Reassure Offer sympathy + support. coped well
Need help.
Respite — & then may want her back = ↑
home help. SS — benefits; aids

YOU ARE NOW APPROXIMATELY HALF WAY THROUGH THIS PAPER

⑤ what are M-in-laws feelings — is she able to give informed consent ? underlying problems c family
Pt autonomy; does she have insight

⑥ Involve son & other children

6. Steven Meade has recently been admitted to the local psychiatric hospital with a diagnosis of schizophrenia. The psychiatrist would like to offer some family therapy and Steven's parents Brian and Julie ask you what this therapy is and what Steven's problems have to do with them. How would you handle this situation?

Breaking Bad news? "Consultation probs"

Invite both to joint consultation? Allow them to express their feelings on recent events.
Ideas, concerns & expectations? Guilt, anxieties, stigma
<u>Acknowledge this confusion</u>

Explain natural Hx of illness — may be de-stigmatise
of — Sx; signs
Δ, Prognosis ; Rx ; FU.

Explain nature of family therapy in simple terms
& effect of family on illness. Negative &
— EE - expressed emotions Don't be accusing
- explain multi-factorial nature of disease

Advise them to go along with Rx & offer

FU for advice + support
? any written literature re: disease

? <u>Hidden agenda</u> — wanting to discuss Stephen
<u>What has already been said by Ψ</u>

<u>Principles of giving information</u> — small amounts ; non-technical
simple ; check for understanding
& opportunity to ask Qu's

? Parents feelings of guilt/blame

7. Paula, aged 22 months, and her 19 year old mother Tessa Bales enter with their health visitor who is concerned that Paula is 'failing to thrive'. What is your role in the further management of this case?

Dealing with other health professionals.
    Problem solving approach
    Views of Mother, HV or doctor — maintain good relations

Allow Paula to express worries + concerns — what
                         — trust + rapport
are here problems ? hidden agenda. Physical /social
or emotional problems — Paula /mother.

Take history — childhood
                — development
                — weights /heights
                — imm :
                — illness /recent
                — dietary hx

Observe child.
Hx from HV — ? hidden agenda ; express her ideas
                                concerns
        — why is she with pt
        — discuss I her at different time
        — look at centile charts

Examine child
        — generally ; specific
: Ix — Baseline bloods /urine /Cxr   ?Δ "FTT"
    — referral in-pt /out-pt
    — child community   Rx — as necessary
    — observe
Allow — follow-up mother /child /HV
Give information in simple terms
Establish shared Mx plan — Tessa, H.V

? Family at risk

8. Tessa seems totally unconcerned by Paula's problems. What are the possible reasons for Tessa's behaviour?

Problems solving.
  Physical ; social ; emotional ; psychological.

Discuss with Tessa /a H.V - what she feels problems
are.

(A) Does she see problems - may think things are O.K
  ? inexperienced mother - poor extended family
      - role models ↓
      - ↓ educated
      - ° comparison - socially isolated

(B) If there are problems, Tessa may not see them
  - (i) Physical problems - in self ; others in family
      - ? An iglandula fever
  (ii) Social - ? poor home conditions - or own ; out all h
                          poor bonding
  time ; disorganised family
      - financially ↓ - unable to afford food
          - spend money elsewhere
      - problems c partner - abuse ; Et-oh ; drug

  (iii) Emotional / psych - depressed ; low IQ
      - personality disorder
      - other psychosis

a/w H.V - she may know her better
  May need to examine Tessa, take history
      and ? admit - mother / baby unit
          - refer SS ; Y ; counselling
          - F.u -c GP / H.V

64 Complex situation

9. Your last patient is Bryan Smedley, a 22 year old unemployed labourer with a fresh wound on his hand. Recently he has been increasingly using heroin and cocaine and admits to cutting his hand during a recent burglary. What issues does this presentation present? Duties to pt & to society

Social problems; Infectious risk ; drug addictions
& known involvement in crime ? confidentiality /ethics

Firstly to assess acute situation — how bad is
wound / bleeding /damage to blood vessels /tendons
— assess in safe area — watch for blood spills → (?confidentility)
— infectious risk — gloves ; inform other staff
If needs A+E R — apply 1st aid → X-R for FB
& suturing & assessment. Give letter informing them
of health risk — infection
If Rx in surgery — check tetanus status +
                            (Confidentiality re burglary + taking drugs)
Rx
    How well do you know him — establish rapport
+ trust.
    Allow him to express his anxieties /problems. —many
social problems, Allow expansion:
    Does he want help with ① Social situation
— alternative to burglary — confidential ∴ will not
tell police — but if danger to self /society may
may feel morally obligated to tell police — down
② Drug addiction? or occasional use — does he want help
to stop — refer to addiction clinic — ∴ have to
let home office know. ↑ risk of other illness
— if IV use — HIV, hep B
feelings/ confidence in self dealing with these problems
                            Doctors safety + practice safety
65

10. During the evening at home the local day release course organiser phones you and asks if you can give a talk on 'Improving care to socially deprived patients'. What areas would you like to cover?

Bad day!   Large, vague subject

Present situation

Ideal situation — what is possible within constraints of NHS OP   Recognise at-risk gp eg Jarman index

Start with history, ? some studies — inverse care law
— those who need care most seek it least

why is this a problems — problems with society/politics/medicine — concentrate on medical side

Doctors —difficulty seeking out those in need
— attitude /class //language difference
— ?approachable
— poor social conditions → ↑ morbidity/mortality

↑ smoking /etoh/ unemployment /diet /↓ uptake of screening
↓ knowledge /contact ē media

Improvements

Make governments aware of problems — they can tackle social inequalities
↑ media campaigns to reach these people
↓ advertising of smoking
Change in doctors training /attitudes
— seek out those in need — advise /follow-up
Talk about own practice — practice profile

66

— medical ; psycholg + social influences
Other agencies -Nursing — team approach — H.V T.S.W
+ voluntary   ? staff training

THE CRITICAL READING QUESTION PAPER

EXAMINATION ADVICE

The Critical Reading Question Paper (CRQ) assesses a candidate's ability to understand, summarise and evaluate published papers and written material encountered in general practice. The ability to apply to general practice what has been read is also tested. The examination is oriented towards general practice in Britain and candidates are advised to concentrate their reading on the reputable books and journals commonly available to British general practitioners. The paper is of 2 hours duration but an additional 15 minutes is allowed for candidates to read the presented material. The paper normally contains three questions, each carrying equal marks. The subject matter covers the areas of health and disease, medicine and society and practice management. Answers should be in expanded note form to allow for the maximum amount of information to be written down in the minimum length of time. The answers should be legible and abbreviations should be avoided since they can be misinterpreted.

Question 1.
Candidates are presented with a published paper from an established medical journal relevant to British general practice and are tested on the ability to recognise the main issues raised, comment where appropriate on the design of the study and discuss the implications and practical application of the results to general practice.

Question 2.
Candidates are examined on their familiarity with published literature in areas of current concern and interest in general practice. Marks are given for demonstrating factual knowledge and quoting references but the majority of marks are awarded to those who show that they have read and understood relevant literature on the subject.

Question 3.
Candidates are presented with written material commonly encountered in general practice and are asked to analyse and respond. For example this may take the form of a letter, a practice protocol, a practice report, practice audit or advertising material. Candidates are expected to demonstrate their ability to analyse the practical implications of the presented material for their work as general practitioners.

The CRQ paper replaced the previous Practice Topic Paper, mainly in an attempt to widen the sampling of the various areas of general practice. Good examination technique is again important and remembering to pace yourself within the time allotted is essential. Each question (including each part of each question) is marked by a different examiner and he/she will have a marking schedule for that question. To generate maximum marks each part of each question should be fully answered – hence the need for good time management. Practice at answering questions in limited time is time well spent.

The basic principles of good exam technique are:
1. Believe in yourself! If the examiners can answer the question, so can you.
2. Read the question and source material carefully. Only answer what you have been asked. It often helps to underline key words. There are no marks for irrelevant information.
3. Make an answer plan.
4. Remember to write legibly.
5. Time yourself and keep within the limits for each question.
6. You will always make mistakes, so allow a minute or so to read through your paper to correct any stupid errors.

The marking of the CRQ is, like the MEQ, based on a consensus 'good answer' generated by a group of examiners. The candidates' answers are assessed by comparison with that of the examiners taking into account the number of issues presented and the depth to which they are discussed. Remember that, if a question asks you to comment, this should include both good and bad points about the study or data.

CRQ PAPER : QUESTION 1

Increasingly we are bombarded with research literature either in published papers or via pharmaceutical company advertising. The ability to assess critically the quality of the studies and their implications for general practice is becoming ever more important. This is the rationale for including this question in the new CRQ. A detailed knowledge of statistics is not required, but awareness of broad concepts is.

Critically assessing a clinical paper can seem a daunting prospect. However, like most other things, with a planned approach it is very straightforward. Don't be put off by the idea that a paper has been published in a journal. You, as a trained professional, are perfectly able to pick out its good and bad points and extract from it any information relevant to your practice.

On reading a paper, a quick way to assess it is to ask yourself if the paper answers the following questions:

What are they trying to do?

Why did they start?

What did they do?

What did they find?

What does it mean?

In order to give you a more detailed framework for critically assessing a paper we will give you a list of what to look for in each section. You may not understand every point given — DON'T WORRY. As long as you are aware of at least half the issues you should be able to give an adequate answer. Don't get bogged down in statistics you don't understand. You should be able to give a good answer without understanding statistical detail if you have a sensible approach. If you do understand the statistics, then go ahead and comment on them.

In the exam you may be required to write your own summary of a given paper. We recommend you use the same format as appears in the BMJ, i.e.

Objective of study
Design of study
Setting of study
Patients studied
Main outcome measures
Results
Conclusions

This format enables you to give a logical and complete answer. Practice summarising articles from the BMJ and College journal. This is a good way to pick up the salient points of a paper, even if you are not asked to do it in the exam itself.

If you would like more information then the following book is recommended:
Research Methods for General Practitioners.
David Armstrong, Michael Calnan, John Grace.
Oxford University Press 1989.

A STRUCTURED APPROACH TO CLINICAL PAPERS

Introduction

Are the aims of the paper stated clearly and unambiguously?

Was there an adequate literature search?

Method

Where and in what situation was the study carried out i.e. the setting. It may be:
- Inner-city
- Rural
- Hospital
- General Practice etc.

Is the sample large enough?

If the study is of an intervention, has a control group (with no intervention) been compared with the study group? If so, have the groups been randomised, and how?

Are the treatment and control groups matched?

Is the time span appropriate? The time allowed must be long enough for the outcome to occur.

For outcomes, what are the criteria? How were they developed? Are they clinically relevant? Are they accurate and reproducible? (Consider the wide variation included in the term 'CVA'.) Would all doctors accept this end-point? Has observer bias been removed?

If studying process of care do the described outcomes depend on that process?

Have all relevant outcomes been reported?

If a questionnaire is used, are the questions clearly phrased? Is an example of the questionnaire shown? Was a pilot study done? Logarithmic scales may have been used to amplify small differences in results — you need to be aware of this.

Results

Is the display of information clear? E.g. good use of graphs, tables, bar charts. Numbers are preferable to percentages. Logarithmic scales may have been used to amplify small differences in results — you need to be aware of this.

Has the statistical analysis been appropriate and accurate?

Is the response rate good? A poor response rate can introduce bias — e.g. only those with a good response to a particular treatment might bother to return a questionnaire.

Have non responders been followed up? This can help to reduce bias.

Have outside factors which may have affected the results been taken into account?

Discussion

Have the initial objectives of the study been reached?

Has the data been interpreted objectively?

Are the inferences drawn supported by data obtained during the study?

Are the results clinically significant?

Are there any conclusions which are not supported by facts? What are these?

Are any results left 'unspoken'? Is there any explanation of why these results are not discussed?

Are there any questions arising from the study which require further evaluation?

Are the results relevant to your own practice? e.g.

— is the study population similar to your own?
— do you have similar procedures?

Are there any implications for your practice and for practice in general?

References

Are the references up to date and relevant?

Overall Impression

Was the presentation of the article clear?
Were the results valid?
Was the study ethical?
Was the study worthwhile?

Further information on clinical papers:

The information below explains some of the terminology used in studies, and some of the statistics used. Use what you understand. You may find it makes more sense after you have read a few papers using the format above.

Types of study

Different types of studies can be done:

1. **Study of structure:** These studies look at physical facilities, e.g. quality of medical records. They are easy to perform but are often no reflection of quality of care.

2. **Study of process:** Looks at the actions and interventions of health professionals and their staff in patient care. E.g. The organisation of an appointment system.

3. **Study of outcome:** Outcome studies consider the end points of health care. Health care should aim to reduce mortality and morbidity rates.

   They are of two main types:

   (a) **Interventions** — The effect of an action on a study group is considered.

   (b) **Correlations** — The characteristics of a group of patients is studied to see if a common factor is associated with a given outcome.

For outcome studies to be reliable, the following are important:

- the outcome described should be accurate and reproducible and not affected by observer bias.

- the sample size must be large enough.

- the study period must be long enough.

- the outcome must be dependent on the intervention being studied.

- if the study uses an intervention, than a control group with no intervention should be compared to the study group.

Methods of study

Cohort study — This identifies 2 groups which are followed to see if there are any differences in outcome. E.g. HRT and non-HRT users are studied, and the incidence of disease in each group compared. The groups should be otherwise matched.

Case control — This is a type of study where a group of patients with a disease is compared to a control group (without the disease) to identify any differences in their characteristics.

Statistical terms

Mode — The result which occurs most often.

Mean — The average i.e. the sum total divided by the number of observations.

Median — The midway value, halfway between the highest and lowest result.

In a normal distribution all three of the above have the same value.

Range — The spread of results from the highest to the lowest.

Standard deviation — This is a measure of the spread around the mean. A calculation from the data produces a value known as the standard deviation (SD).
In a normal distribution: 65% of the values lie within 1 SD
95% "   "   "   "   "   2 SD
99% "   "   "   "   "   3 SD

Descriptive data — i.e. summarised and presented in a meaningful form (e.g. tables and graphs).

Inferential statistics — These are more difficult to understand for the statistically unaware. The basis of inferential statistics is that inferences are drawn from mathematical theories of probabilities.

Usually the 'Null Hypothesis' is being tested. This assumes that there is an even chance of either success or failure occurring. The method is used to see if any observed effect is due to a particular intervention and whether this effect happens more often than would be expected by chance. If so, it is said to be 'statistically significant'.

p value — This is a common expression to measure statistical significance. The accepted level of 'significance' is p, i.e. there is a 5% (1 in 20) or less likelihood that the event has occurred by chance.

We usually assume that the paper has been reviewed by a statistician to ensure that the statistical measure used is appropriate. This may not be the case and using a sensible approach it is often easy to find quite basic faults.

Questionnaire design

Many papers include the use of a questionnaire. Essential points to look for include:

a) Use of user-friendly questions — the questions should be easy to understand in terms of reading age and phrasing. (The average reading age for many tabloid newspapers is 12.)

b) Mid point bias — This means that people are more likely to choose the middle value when given an odd number of alternatives. Giving an even number of alternatives allows for greater discrimination between answers.

c) Whether the questionnaire was piloted to see if it was appropriate

d) Is there a statement of how much the response is intention or actual behaviour? We all know how pre-election surveys of intention to vote can be erroneous.

Using the basic checklist as a framework will enable you to answer the questions adequately. A detailed knowledge of statistics will only gain you a few extra marks.

INSTRUCTIONS FOR THE CRQ PAPER
(i.e. Questions 1, 2 & 3)

1. You are advised to read the relevant questions before reading the presented material.

2. Each part carries equal marks.

3. Answers should be in expanded note form unless you are specifically instructed otherwise. The total time allowed is two and a quarter hours. You are advised to spend at least fifteen minutes carefully reading the presented material and equal time on each of the question parts.

4. Each page is marked by a different examiner. You should therefore give a complete answer to each question **even if this involves repetition of part of an earlier answer.**

5. Answers should be written in the space provided. If more room is required use the reverse side of the question sheet.

6. In question 2 you will gain marks when mentioning current literature by describing its contribution to the arguments which you are presenting and, where appropriate, commenting on its credibility. If possible you should indicate the source and approximate year of publication of material referred to in your answer. Merely listing references will not suffice. The majority of marks are awarded for stating the current views on the topic.

INSTRUCTIONS:

1. Summarise the following article.

2. Comment on the design of the study and the presentation of the results (method and results section of the paper).

3. If the conclusions of this paper were supported by further research what are the implications for you as a general practioner?

Can health screening damage your health?

H.G. Stoate, MSc, MRCGP, general practitioner

Reprinted with the kind permission of the *Journal of the Royal College of General Practitioners, 1989*

Introduction

ADULT screening for coronary risk factors in general practice is widely advocated on the grounds that it can save lives or at least reduce morbidity. Furthermore, it is believed that making people aware of risk factors will enable them to exert greater control over their own health. Advocates of screening tend to assume that there are only two possible outcomes of screening: benefit or no effect. A third possibility, harm, is frequently ignored. It can be argued that the debate about who to screen and for what conditions should be widened to take more account of its effect on a person's mental state and subsequent behaviour.

In order for screening to be of benefit it must be capable of detecting disease or potential disease not only before its usual clinical presentation but also before the point at which intervention becomes ineffective, sometimes called the 'critical point'.[1] Unfortunately, relatively few medical conditions satisfy these criteria,[2] and this may be one reason why many studies of adult health screening have had disappointing results. The Kaiser Permanente study[3] failed to prove the case for multiphasic screening as opposed to conventional care. The authors of the south east London screening study found no good evidence of the usefulness of screening in middle-aged adults. Their conclusions were unequivocal: 'We believe that the use of general practice based multiphasic screening in the middle-aged can no longer be advocated on scientific, ethical or economic grounds as a desirable public health measure'.[4] The World Health Organization's European heart study showed no clear effect of screening on coronary heart disease end-points.[5] Even the multiple risk factor intervention trial which looked at high risk men aged bet-ween 25–57 years, found no difference between 'special interven-tion care' and the usual community care over a seven-year period.[6]

These trials all looked at hard end-points such as death or non-fatal myocardial infarction. None looked at the effect of screening programmes on the psychological state and behaviour of the participants. It has been shown by Haynes and colleagues[7] that the labelling of previously undiagnosed hypertensives, detected by screening in the work place, results in increased absenteeism from work. It is therefore known that detecting abnormalities may have significant costs to the patient. What has not been studied is whether there are similar costs to people who do not have risk factors for disease.

This longitudinal controlled study in general practice looked at the effect of a by-invitation screening clinic on the psychological wellbeing of people found to have no detected abnormality, and thus labelled 'normal'. It was hypothesized that screening may make people more aware of illness thus increas-ing their psychological distress.

Method

The study was carried out in a new purpose-built six-handed practice in Bexleyheath, Kent. The practice employs a full-time preventive health worker who runs a by-invitation coronary risk screening clinic for men and women aged between 35 and 65 years. All patients in year of birth cohorts from the age–sex register were invited to make an appointment for a free health check.

The indicator of subjective psychological wellbeing used in this study was the 30 item version of Goldberg's general health questionnaire, a self-administered instrument which measures recent psychological distress, largely ignoring stable personali-ty traits.[8] It is ideal for general practice use,[9] is simple to score[10] and has been shown to be sensitive to change over time.[11] Sub-jects are usually considered to be minor psychiatric 'cases' if they score above the cut-off score of 5.[12] Although the instru-ment is designed to measure psychological distress, it has been shown to correlate with perceived health status.[13]

Housing tenure was used as an indicator of social class.[14] People were classified as living in owner-occupied, council rented or private rented accommodation. This information is obtain-ed with a single question and is particularly useful in postal ques-tionnaires.[15] Previous studies have compared it favourably with the Registrar General's classification, and with socioeconomic group.[16]

Between September 1987 and April 1988 attenders at the screening clinic were handed a general health questionnaire on arrival and asked to complete it before screening. Patients were then screened by the nurse who took a history of smoking, drinking, diet and family history of ischaemic heart disease. Blood pressure, height and weight were measured and urinalysis was performed. Blood was taken for lipids or liver function tests if appropriate. Any risk factors detected were discussed and advice and leaflets given if necessary. To look at the effect of screening on 'healthy' adults, patients found to have any of the following were excluded from the study: previously undetected blood pressure above 160/95 mmHg, newly detected glycosuria, fasting total cholesterol above 6.5 mM, or any other previously undetected abnormality which in the nurse's opinion required referral to the patient's doctor for further action.

Controls were randomly selected from the age–sex register using uninvited years of birth as close as possible to the study group, thus matching fairly closely for age. This group was sent a general health questionnaire by post with a letter asking for their help in a health survey. Reminders were sent after 10 days.

Subjects and controls were contacted in monthly batches of similar size in order to eliminate any seasonal effect on general health questionnaire score. This was achieved by selecting a larger control than subject group. It was reasoned that age–sex registers have a margin of error (10.5% in this case) and that response rates would be inevitably lower for a control group who gain no personal benefit from replying.

Subjects and controls both received a second general health questionnaire by post three months after the first, again with an explanatory covering letter. Reminders were sent to non-responders 10 days later.

Results

During the study period 234 people attended the screening clinic: 15 people (6.4%) were found to have previously undetected abnormalities and were therefore excluded from the study; two patients were in the process of moving house and two refused to take part; 215 patients were therefore enrolled. A total of 255 control patients were selected: three had been previously screened and 27 were unknown at their registered address; 225 controls were therefore included in the study. These were thus matched for age not sex. Interestingly, however, the groups had very similar sex ratios, indicating that there was no sex bias in attending for screening.

Response rates for the two questionnaires are shown in Table 1. The response rate of the control group to both questionnaires was lower than the study group. There was a close similarity in housing tenure between the study and control groups (Table 2). The sex ratios of the two groups were also similar with women comprising 56.6% of the study and 57.4% of control groups ($\chi^2 = 0.049$, not significant).

Table 1. Response rates for the two questionnaires.

		Number (%) of patients	
	Enrolled	Completed first questionnaire	Completed first and second questionnaire
Study group	215	215 *(100.0)*	189 *(87.9)*
Controls	225	185 *(82.2)*	155 *(68.8)*

Table 2. Housing tenure of respondents.

	Number (%) of respondents		
	Owner occupied	Council rented	Private rented
Study group (n = 189)	172 *(91.0)*	12 *(6.3)*	5 *(2.6)*
Control group (n = 155)	138 *(89.0)*	10 *(6.4)*	7 *(4.5)*

Owner occupied versus rented (private + council), $\chi^2 = 0.33$, df = 1, not significant.

When the general health questionnaire scores were compared for the two groups there were two important results. First, significantly fewer of those attending for screening had psychological distress on the first questionnaire than the control group (χ^2 with Yates' correction = 6.09, df = 1, $P<0.05$). Secondly, significantly more of the screened group had a high general health questionnaire score three months after screening than before (Table 3). The control group showed a non-significant fall in general health questionnaire score during the three-month period.

Discussion

The study demonstrated a significant increase in psychological distress in healthy adults who have been screened for coronary heart disease risk factors. An association, however, does not prove causation — the effect may be due to selection or artefact — and it is important to address some of the weaknesses of the study design.

It is unfortunate that a smaller proportion of the control patients completed both questionnaires, despite a postal reminder, but it was felt to be important to avoid personal contact

Table 3. Study and control group respondents with general health questionnaire (GHQ) scores of 5 or more.

	Percentage of respondents scoring >5 (95% confidence intervals)		
	First GHQ	Second GHQ	Chi-squared test with Yates' correction
Study group (n = 189)	21.7 (15.2–26.8)	35.4 (28.2–41.8)	$\chi^2 = 8.10$, df = 1, P<0.01
Control group (n = 155)	34.1 (26.6–41.4)	25.8 (18.0–32.0)	$\chi^2 = 2.21$, df = 1, NS

by telephone in case this influenced the scores. The fact that fewer of those attending for screening had high initial general health questionnaire scores than the control group needs to be considered. It might be argued that anxious people or those with real or imagined health problems will be more likely to accept an invitation for screening. If so, we could expect a higher proportion of patients with high initial general health questionnaire scores, rather than the reverse. Attenders for screening are self-selected and certainly likely to be different from a random group of patients with similar socioeconomic variables. The reasons why psychologically healthier people attend for screening is interesting and further work is planned to study this.

The decrease in scores for the control groups between the first and second questionnaires is the usual result seen with repeat administration of the general health questionnaire.[8] What was totally unexpected was that significantly more of the study group had scores indicating psychological distress after screening than before. A study design can only eliminate known dependent variables and the higher general health questionnaire scores in the subject group may be a reflection of unknown variables. It is unlikely, however, that this could entirely explain significant differences between two fairly well matched groups. The possibility of a direct causal relationship between screening and increased stress cannot be ignored.

It is interesting to speculate about the nature of this relationship. The impression given by some patients was that receiving a letter warning them of risk factors for coronary disease and premature death made them feel that they had been negligent. This type of systematic screening may have made some people more aware of their mortality and, more hypochondriacal, leading to greater psychological distress. If patients become more dependent on health services to deal with their life problems this has serious implications, not only for patients themselves but for the health services. General practitioners are being encouraged to screen more but Kleinman[17] warned that as 90% of episodes of illness are dealt with without resort to the doctor, a shift of only 10% in the proportion presenting to general practitioners would double our workload.

More work is needed in this area. Given that we have as yet no conclusive proof that screening alters the natural history of disease in a significant proportion of those screened,[2,18] we must be cautious in our appraisal of measures which appear to reduce risk factors by detection and intervention. As Rose and Barker put it,[19] 'The outcome of screening must be judged in terms of its effect on mortality and illness and not in terms of its restoration of biochemical or other test results, to normal'. We must also address the possibility, previously largely ignored, that for some people at least, screening can do more harm than good.

References

1. Sackett D, Haynes R, Tugwell P. *Clinical epidemiology.* Boston: Little Brown, 1985.
2. Cochrane A, Holland W. Validation of screening procedures. *Br Med Bull* 1971; **27**: 3-8.
3. Collen MF, Dales LG, Friedman GD, *et al.* Multiphasic checkup evaluation study 4. *Prev Med* 1973; **2**: 236-246.
4. South east London study group. A controlled trial of multiphasic screening in middle age. Results of the south east London screening study. *Int J Epidemiol* 1977; **6**: 357-363.
5. Rose G, Tunstall-Pedoe H, Heller R. The UK heart disease prevention project. Incidence and mortality results. *Lancet* 1983; **1**: 1062-1065.
6. Multiple risk factor intervention trial research group. The multiple risk factor intervention trial. *JAMA* 1982; **248**: 1465-1477.
7. Haynes R, Sackett D, Taylor D, *et al.* Increased absenteeism from work after detection and labelling of hypertensive patients. *N Engl J Med* 1978; **299**: 741-744.
8. Goldberg D. *Manual of the general health questionaire.* Windsor: NFER-Nelson, 1978.
9. Goldberg D, Blackwell B. Psychiatric illness in general practice. *Br Med J* 1970; **2**: 439-443.
10. Goldberg D, Huxley P. *Mental illness in the community.* London: Tavistock, 1980.
11. Goldberg D. *The detection of psychiatric illness by questionnaire.* Oxford University Press, 1972.
12. Goldberg D. *Users guide to the general health questionnaire.* Windsor: NFER-Nelson (in press).
13. Tessler R, Mechanic D. Psychological distress and perceived health status. *J Health Soc Behaviour* 1978; **19**: 254-262.

14. Morgan M. Measuring social inequalities. Occupational classifications and their alternatives. *Community Med* 1983; **5:** 116-124.
15. Marsh C. Social class and occupation. In: Burgess R (ed). *Key variables in social investigation.* London: Routledge and Kegan Paul, 1986.
16. Goldblatt P, Fox A. Household morbidity from the OPCS longitudinal study. *Population Trends* 1978; **14:** 20-27.
17. Kleinman A, Eisenberg L, Good B. Culture, illness and care. *Ann Intern Med* 1978; **88:** 251-259.
18. D'Souza M. Early diagnosis and multiphasic screening; In: Bennett A (ed). *Recent advances in community medicine.* Edinburgh: Churchill Livingstone, 1978.
19. Rose G, Barker D. *Epidemiology for the uninitiated.* London: British Medical Association, 1986.

INSTRUCTIONS:

1. Summarise the article attached.

2. Comment on the design of the study and the presentation of the results (method and results section of the paper).

3. If the conclusions of this paper were supported by further research what are the implications for you as a general practioner?

Survey of general practitioners' advice for travellers to Turkey

V. Usherwood, SRN, research sister and T.P. Underwood, MRCP, MRCGP, research fellow, Department of General Practice, University of Glasgow.

Reprinted with the kind permission of the *Journal of the Royal College of General Practitioners, 1989*

Introduction

DURING a recent family holiday in Turkey, the authors were surprised by the variety of preventive care measures that had been offered to fellow travellers. These ranged from advice that no particular health precautions were necessary, through the provision of antimalarials alone, to antimalarial medication with immunization against typhoid, cholera, tetanus, poliomyelitis and hepatitis A.

Reid and colleagues reviewed the health advice contained in 64 travel brochures[1] and identified substantial inadequacies and inconsistencies in the information provided. Although many prospective tourists consult their doctors for advice no survey of the advice given by general practitioners to foreign travellers appears to have been carried out. It was therefore decided to survey the advice that doctors in Inverclyde, a district of Strathclyde, would offer a patient planning a package holiday in a popular resort in western Turkey.

Method

In June/July 1988 60 of the 62 principals practising in Inverclyde were sent a self-administered questionnaire seeking details of the advice that they would typically offer a generally healthy unmarried young man, with no relevant past medical history or known allergies, who was planning a package holiday in Turkey. It was explained that the patient and three friends would be staying for two weeks in an apartment in Bodrum, an increasingly popular resort on the west (Aegean) coast of the country.

The general practitioners were asked to describe their normal practice, rather than to provide model answers in response to each question. Although the questionnaires were identified by a serial number, an undertaking was given that this would be used only to identify non-responders and to identify those respondents who requested a copy of the tabulated results of the survey, and not to match answers to individual doctors.

Two weeks after the questionnaires were first distributed, a further copy with a reminder letter was sent to each of the non-responders.

The questionnaire asked the respondents to list immunizations and other prophylactic medication that they would recommend to the young man, and to indicate their own sources of guidance, if any, in their answers to the question. They were also asked what other advice they would offer the traveller concerning the proposed trip. Three final questions asked whether the doctors had been consulted for travel advice by patients visiting Turkey during 1988, whether the doctors had visited Turkey themselves, and whether they required a copy of the tabulated results of the survey.

Results

Table 1. Prophylaxis that would be recommended by the 50 general practitioners to a tourist planning a package holiday in Bodrum, Turkey.

Prophylaxis	Number (%) of GPs recommending prophylaxis	DHSS advice[a]
Typhoid immunization	48 (*96*)	Recommended
Cholera immunization	39 (*78*)	Recommended
Polio immunization	37 (*74*)	Recommended
Malaria prophylaxis	26 (*52*)	Ambiguous
Tetanus immunization[c]	23 (*46*)	Not recommended
Human normal immunoglobulin[c]	6 (*12*)	Not recommended
Diphtheria immunization	1 (*2*)	Not recommended

[a]Leaflet SA40, reference 2. [b]Recommended in table on page 13 but not recommended on map on page 6. [c]Leaflet SA40 recommends tetanus immunization only for areas where medical facilities are not readily available, and human normal immunoglobulin in places where sanitation is primitive. Bodrum is not covered by these descriptions.[3]

Fifty (83%) of the 60 general practitioners returned a completed questionnaire. Forty one of the respondents (82%) had been consulted for travel advice by prospective visitors to Turkey during 1988, and five (10%) had visited the country themselves. The immunizations and other prophylactics that the respondents would offer to the young man are listed in Table 1. For comparison, the current Department of Health and Social Security advice contained in leaflet SA40[2] is also tabulated. This leaflet had been distributed by the local health board to all the principals in this study a few months before the survey. Ignoring any advice given concerning antimalarials about which the leaflet is equivocal, only 18 of the respondents (36%) would offer exactly the advice contained in the leaflet. However, all of the doctors would offer some prophylactic medication. Although the tourist would be more likely to receive recommended prophylactics than those not recommended, there were some discrepancies.

The source or sources of guidance that the doctors claimed to have consulted before they answered the question on prophylaxis are recorded in Table 2. Thirty six of the respondents consulted some source, and in 34 cases it was possible to compare the advice given by the doctor with the guidance provided by the source. Only 11 of the doctors gave the tourist exactly the advice provided in the source consulted.

Table 2. Sources of guidance consulted by the 50 general practitioners before deciding on prophylactic advice.

Source	Number (%) of GPs consulting source
Weekly medical newspaper[a]	24 *(48)*
Monthly index of medical specialities	7 *(14)*
Communicable Diseases (Scotland) Unit	6 *(12)*
British national formulary	2 *(4)*
DHSS leaflet SA40[b]	2 *(4)*
Local pharmacy	1 *(2)*
Local travel agency	1 *(2)*
No source consulted	14 *(28)*

[a]Vaccination chart, *Doctor* 1988; 30 June: 48. Foreign travel guide, *Pulse* 1988; 2 July: 51. [b]Reference 2.

Table 3. Health advice that would be offered by the 50 general practitioners.

Topic of advice	Number (%) of GPs who would raise topic
Care with food or water	35 *(70)*
Risks of excessive exposure to sun	15 *(30)*
Safe sex practices	9 *(18)*
Avoidance of insect bites	4 *(8)*
Danger of rabies	3 *(6)*
Dangers of illicit drug use	2 *(4)*
Health insurance	2 *(4)*
Advisory leaflet given	2 *(4)*

Table 3 lists the health advice that the doctors claimed that they would offer. Apart from the advice to take care over food or water, none of the topics listed was mentioned by more than a third of the respondents. In contrast, all the topics are considered in one or other of DHSS leaflets SA40[2] and SA41.[4]

Thirty eight of the respondents (76%) requested a copy of the tabulated results of the survey.

Discussion

Prophylactic medication and immunization for foreign travel fall into two categories. Certain immunizations may be required by the countries visited, but the Turkish authorities place no such imposition on visitors from the UK at present. Other prophylactics may be recommended by the DHSS or expert medical opinion, but are not legal requirements. The problem facing general practitioners is in defining the recommendations for an individual patient and this is exacerbated by the varying opinions contained in the sources of expert guidance.

The discrepancy concerning malaria prophylaxis in leaflet SA40[2] is mirrored elsewhere. The vaccination chart in *Doctor* (30 June 1988) recommends antimalarials for travellers to western Turkey, while the foreign travel guide in *Pulse* (2 July 1988) and the *Monthly index of medical specialities* refer to a seasonal risk. At the time of the study the Ross Institute 24-hour tape service advised that malaria prophylaxis was not currently required in western Turkey.

Similar confusion exists over immunizations. Although all the sources referred to in Table 2 recommend typhoid and cholera immunizations, doubt has been expressed about the need for cholera immunization[5] and the Joint Committee on Vaccination and Immunization[6] merely states that typhoid immunization should be considered. However, immunization of a traveller to Turkey against typhoid attracts a fee for National Health Service general practitioners, whereas immunization against cholera does not.[7]

Human normal immunoglobulin was recommended in the *Pulse* foreign travel guide but nowhere else, although a case can be made for this for all tourists seronegative for hepatitis A.[10]

Doctors are used to sifting a wide range of guidance on a problem, then drawing a conclusion. However, the variation contained in the sources described here is less than ideal. Such disagreement between experts is to be expected where their advice is based on imprecise epidemiological data, and on partly subjective assessment of the risks and benefits of immunization. However, the lack of consensus is unhelpful to the non-expert practitioner. This may be one reason for the discrepancies between the source consulted and the advice offered by 23 doctors. Certainly it seems likely that the range of guidance provided to general practitioners was responsible for the variation between respondents. At best, this variation will reduce patients' confidence in their doctor's advice. At worst, some tourists will travel without adequate protection, or will receive unnecessary injections.

The health advice that would be offered by most of the respondents is disappointing but probably reflects the limited time available during a routine consultation. Furthermore, most general practitioners are aware that patients take away only a small proportion of the advice given, so that covering all the topics listed in Table 3 would probably be counter productive. Nevertheless, advice given in a doctor's surgery carries special weight[11] and a useful opportunity for health promotion may have been missed.

The method used in this study has its limitations as the responses could not be validated against the doctors' actual practice. Although care was taken to encourage the respondents to describe their normal practice, the answers that they gave were probably more complete and received more consideration than is sometimes possible during a busy surgery.

Two conclusions can be drawn from this study: patients do not receive consistent advice on prophylaxis from different doctors, and little other health advice is offered to travellers during consultations. Although there is clearly no single correct set of guidelines for general practitioners, it would help if the sources of advice that do exist agreed with each other. The routine annual supply of a reasonable number of copies of leaflets SA40[2] and SA41[4] to all general practitioners would provide useful literature for tourists when they consult, and leaflet SA41 might also be included with airline tickets. The problem of illness associated with travel is not small; one review showed an overall attack rate of 47% in a sample of over 4000 travellers.[12]

References

1. Reid D, Cossar JH, Ako TI, Dewar RD. Do travel brochures give adequate advice on avoiding illness? *Br Med J* 1986; **293**: 1472.
2. Department of Health and Social Security. *Before you go (SA40)*. London: HMSO, 1988.
3. Brosnahan T. *Turkey, a travel survival kit*. 2nd edition. South Yarra, Australia: Lonely Planet, 1988.

4. Department of Health and Social Security. *While you're away (SA41).* London: HMSO, 1988

5. Morger H, Steffen R, Schar M. Epidemiology of cholera in travellers, and conclusions for vaccination recommendations. *Br Med J* 1983; **286:** 184-186.

6. Joint Committee on Vaccination and Immunization. *Immunization against infectious disease.* London: HMSO, 1988.

7. Scottish Home and Health Department. *Statement of fees and allowances payable to general medical practitioners in Scotland.* Edinburgh: SHHD.

8. Frame PS. A critical review of adult health maintenance. Part 2. Prevention of infectious diseases *J Fam Pract* 1986; **22:** 417-422.

9. Howie JGR. Anyone for tetanus? *Br Med J* 1988; **297:** 570-571.

10. Cossar JH, Reid D. Not all travellers need immunoglobulin for hepatitis A. *Br Med J* 1987; **294:** 1503.

11. Fowler G. General practice and health promotion. In: Smith GT (ed). *Health, education and general practice.* London: Office of Health Economics, 1985: 18-20.

12. Cossar JH, Reid D, Grist NR, *et al.* Illness associated with travel. A ten year review. *Travel Medicine International* 1985; **3:** 13-18.

CRQ PAPER : QUESTION 2

This question is very similar to the old style Practice Topic Question. However, remember it is only one section of the CRQ paper and so you are only allowed 40 minutes to answer it.

Revision planning for this question consists of systematically working through the revision 'hot topics', as discussed in the chapter on Revision Planning. Detailed references are not required. However, candidates should be aware of the names of important studies e.g. MRFIT (Multiple Risk Factor Intervention Trial). Editorials and leading articles in the British Medical Journal and The British Journal of General Practice often provide excellent reviews of current important areas.

Remember the instructions to candidates:
- In question 2 you will gain marks when mentioning current literature by describing its contribution to the arguments which you are presenting and, where appropriate, commenting on its credibility.
- If possible you should indicate the source and approximate year of publication of material referred to in your answer.
- Merely listing references will not suffice.
- The majority of marks are awarded for clearly stating the current views on the topic.

For example:

Question 2A: Outline current thinking on first line drug treatment for mild to moderate hypertension.

Question 2B: Outline and evaluate recent evidence supporting longer consultations in general practice.

Question 2C: Discuss the evidence concerning the role of antibiotics in treating otitis media in children.

This should not be too difficult if one remembers that the questions for the summer and winter exam are set, and the marking schedules generated, at the annual examiners' meeting which is held in March or April of that year. Successful revision thus requires a thorough literature review of the previous one to two years. However, reading should not stop at the April issues! You will probably be asked about more recent topics in the oral examination.

CRQ PAPER : QUESTION 3

For this question a similar answering technique to that of the MEQ paper is helpful. Lateral thinking about problems is certainly an important skill, as is the ability to analyse information.

Sample Question A:

PRACTICE ANNUAL REPORT

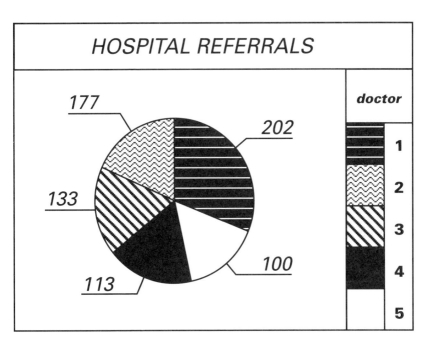

1. Comment on the above data.

2. What are the possible causes of variation in hospital referrals made by each doctor?

Sample Question B:

Somerset House
Private Consulting Suite
Rich Town

Dear Dr,

I saw Mr X today. He arrived at my rooms without a letter. I contacted your surgery to check it was in order for me to see him. He saw his optician last week who noted optic pressures of 19 and 20. I confirmed these today. He has full visual fields. I feel it is sufficient at present to keep him under review and have transferred him to my NHS list for this.

Kind regards,

Mr Pompous

1. What issues are raised?

2. List the advantages and disadvantages of open referral.

Sample Question C:

ASTHMA PROTOCOL

1. Word 'asthma' to be written on top of notes.
2. Indexed in disease register.
3. Treat energetically in the chronic phase with a ß stimulant.
4. Encourage patients always to have medication in reserve.
5. Allow practice nurse to use nebuliser before being seen by the doctor. Must have pre- and post-peak flow rates.
6. Nebuliser not to be used more than 4 hourly by patients and not longer than 24 hours without a review by doctor.
7. If little or no response with nebuliser and asthma severe — admission to hospital.
8. If in doubt use crash course of steroids early.
9. Practice nurse to give leaflet regarding asthma.
10. One nebuliser must stay on surgery premises at all times.
11. Inhaled steroids not to be considered in children.

List recommendations for improving the asthma protocol, giving your reasons.

THE ORAL EXAMINATIONS

Candidates who are successful or borderline in the written part of the examination (obtaining 40% or more) will be called to the College for the Oral Examination. This consists of two parts, each lasting 30 minutes. The first oral will be devoted to questioning the candidate on his Practice Experience Questionnaire (PEQ) and the second oral is concerned with answering questions on topics not covered in the first oral.

It is worth noting that being called for the oral does not necessarily mean that you have passed the written exam. It could mean that you have a borderline pass but if you score sufficiently well on the viva it could pull you through the exam as a whole.

Each oral is taken by two examiners and is designed to test knowledge, skills and attitudes. It is a very flexible exam enabling examiners to explore the range and depth of a candidate's abilities. The examiners aim to cover the following seven areas during each oral.

1. **Problem definition**
   Application of knowledge
   Recognition of the whole problem
   Consideration of options and their relative probabilities

2. **Management**
   Whole patient care
   Life threatening problems
   Chronic disease
   Psychological problems
   Use of resources (in the widest sense)
   Prescribing

3. **Prevention**
   Preventive medicine
   Health education

4. **Practice organisation**
   Accessibility
   Team work
   Time management
   Priorities

5. **Communication**
   Doctor-patient communication
   Patients' health beliefs

6. **Professional values**
   Respect for life
   Responsibility and reliability
   Respect for people
   Empathy and sensitivity
   Integrity and ethics

7. **Personal and professional growth**
   Self-awareness
   Balance between personal and professional life
   Self-assessment
   Reading and literature
   Continuing education

Candidates often worry whether the oral is valid and reliable. Great care is taken to ensure these concerns are answered:

1. Each examiner marks each topic independently and gives his own overall assessment. The examiners do not have the results of the written paper available.

2. If candidates are borderline their performance is discussed taking into account their marks in the written papers.

3. All examiners are practising GPs.

4. Examiners are regularly videotaped to appraise their examination technique.

5. At the beginning of the first day of each oral, all examiners mark a standard 'calibration videotape' enabling the examiners to standardise their own marking before they begin.

At the end of the orals each candidate's total mark is calculated and those with passes are informed by post.

ORAL 1

During the first oral the candidate is questioned in detail about his practice and clinical work. This is done by asking questions based on the Practice Experience Questionnaire (PEQ) which will already have been filled in by the candidate and returned to the College.

The PEQ is A4 in size and consists of a practice profile and a record of 25 consecutive patients (including visits) filled in by the candidate. See sample PEQ Appendix 3.

Each candidate should bring with him to the oral a copy of his own submitted PEQ since this can prove a useful *aide memoire*.

It is essential that the candidate has a thorough knowledge of all the patients presented in the diary and particular attention should be paid to presenting features, your definition of the problems, the criteria by which you arrived at a diagnosis and your management. It is quite likely that the examiners will spend 15 minutes on the practice profile and 15 minutes on the record of consecutive patients.

This can be an ideal opportunity for the candidate to score marks since it is one of the rare occasions when he should know more about the patient than the examiner! If you feel a case may present difficulties in discussion, be sure to leave it out of your diary. If you do not, it will probably be the first one seized upon by the examiner. If you mention drug treatment, be sure you know generic names, doses and side effects.

Work load and practice organisation

Be prepared to compare your own practice with the average practice and to explain why it differs e.g. why there are more home visits. You may also be asked to explain practice policies. A useful reference for details on the average practice can be found in *NHS Data Book* by Fry J. and Brooks D. 1985 MTP Press.

Be prepared to discuss:

Special clinics   e.g. diabetic (justify advantages and disadvantages)
Attached staff   e.g. role of psychologists, dietitians, social workers
Premises   e.g. owner-occupied versus rented health centre
Special equipment   e.g. use of nebuliser or ECG.

25 consecutive patients

You are allowed to take an aide memoire into the exam and the patients should be numbered as you submitted them in the PEQ.

The examiner will scan your cases and pick out several for discussion; a particular case may be discussed in depth but often the case merely acts as a stimulus for discussion around a particular topic. The approach described in the section on the MEQ paper can be helpful in preparing for likely questions and so can self questioning e.g. :

What did I do?
How did I do it?
Why did I do it?
How else could I have handled the situation?

This leads to effective problem solving skills on which the examiner will want to concentrate.

Suggested plan:

1. Hypothesis formation. This takes into account a full history, examination, the patient's ideas, concerns and expectations regarding his illness.

2. How the hypotheses were proved or refuted.

3. Investigations, taking into account the financial cost, effect on patient and benefit expected.

4. Working out final diagnosis.

5. Appropriate management plan considering the physical, psychological and social factors contributing to the patient's illness. For drugs used be willing to name dose, side effects, precautions and contraindications.

6. Use of Primary Health Care Team e.g. Health Visitor

7. Referral. Be able to discuss advantages and disadvantages and outcome expected.

8. Long-term care and follow up.

The examiner will often try to link your theoretical knowledge and stated behaviour or management plan to that of a particular patient. This technique is to see if you practice what you preach! If you come unstuck be truthful — the awareness of why you did not follow a particular approach is important.

From the Practice Experience Questionnaire (PEQ) it can be seen that there is increasing emphasis on audit. The College has rightly supported audit as a method of improving quality of care and as a proven method of continuing medical education. However some candidates have a poor awareness of even the basic concepts. A review is enclosed as Appendix 3.

ORAL 2

At the end of the first oral a list of subjects discussed is given to the second set of examiners to avoid repetition.

This is a very flexible part of the examination during which a wide variety of topics can be covered especially those revealing the attitudes of the candidate to his work. Think beforehand how you might answer questions on the topics listed below and interrogate yourself as to why you approach issues in the way you do.

The cases are probably those which the examiners have seen in their own surgeries so they have already worked through the issues raised. They are looking for common sense and competence in decision-making not obscure medical knowledge.

Typical topics

1. Attitudes:
    Patient requests a second opinion. What do you say?
    Patient is abusive to surgery staff.
    Patient demands a home visit for a minor complaint.
    Wife asks you not to tell her husband that he has cancer.
    Use of self help groups.
    Self referral to consultants.
    Patient wanting homoeopathic treatment for illness.
    Patient asking for a full check-up.
    Patient demands slimming tablets.

2. Management plans for common problems.
    Take into account physical, psychological and social factors. Prepare by thinking prior to the exam 'how and why do I manage a particular condition?' e.g.
    snuffles in a baby
    chronic cough in a 2 year old child
    repeated otitis media in 5 year old child
    diarrhoea in 80 year old living alone.

3. Common problems presented:

    a) A 32 year old asymptomatic solicitor has a routine cervical smear. The report reads 'Dyskaryotic cells present. Repeat 6 months'.

        What do you say to her?
        What is your plan for follow up?

    b) Miss Smith, a 22 year old student nurse, comes to the surgery and asks you to destroy all notes concerning her recent abortion.

        How would you respond to her request?

    c) What are the main needs of the terminally ill?

        How do you assess and provide them?
        Who should lead the team that is looking after a dying patient?

    d) A mother brings a 5 year old girl to see you because she has failed a recent hearing test at school.

        How do you manage this problem?
        What are your criteria for referral to an ENT surgeon?

In both orals, the examiners are looking for evidence of a reasonable base of clinical knowledge relating to everyday problems, evidence of the candidate's problem solving ability and for signs that his attitudes to patients and their problems are fitting to general practice. It is probably true that at the root of every decision-making process we undertake, there lies an attitude of which we may not be fully aware. The examiners will be trying to tease this out. One of the commonest questions is 'why do you think that', or 'why did you do that?' Do not be shaken if you are sure that you are right.

Increasingly, you will be asked to justify your approaches with reference to published articles and evidence of reading. This should not be difficult if you have revised in a systematic manner. The MRCGP exam is the only postgraduate exam without a clinical component, although many clinical skills are already tested in the MEQ paper and orals. Currently there is a working party looking at introducing a clinical component into the exam, the exact method to be used is yet to be determined. Whatever method is introduced, emphasis will be placed on an understanding and practical application of the consultation process. This important area is covered in Appendix 2.

Often, there may be no right or wrong answer. You are simply being asked to demonstrate that your course of action was an appropriate one. Questions will tend to be broad and open ended. Closed questions will be used in an attempt to shut you up! The ability to organise and explain one's reasoning and actions is one of the real benefits which come from having successfully undertaken this examination.

ANSWERS AND TEACHING NOTES

ANSWERS TO THE MCQ PRACTICE EXAM

1:True 2:False 3:True 4:False 5:False
A low-fibre diet is thought to predispose to gallstones. 10-30% of all stones are radio-opaque. Medical therapy with chenodeoxycholic acid or ursodeoxycholic acid is effective in more than 50% of patients with cholesterol stones and a functioning gall-bladder.

6:False 7:False 8:True 9:False 10:True
The incidence of Crohn's disease is increasing. Large bowel involvement is more common in the elderly. Erythema nodosum may be associated, but not often enough to help you make the diagnosis. Fatty liver, portal fibrosis and gallstones are all associated.

11:True 12:True 13:True 14:True 15:True
All of the above can cause pruritus ani.

16:True 17:True 18:True 19:True 20:True
The system of statutory notification was created to facilitate the local control of infectious diseases, and also provide information for national surveillance. Medical practitioners should notify the names and addresses of people recognised as, or suspected of, having any of the specified illnesses. Despite significant under-notification, the system provides valuable information on trends in disease incidence.

21:True 22:False 23:False 24:True 25:True
The mode is a particular value with the highest relative frequency, the mean is the average value and the median is the midway value.

26:True 27:True 28:False 29:False 30:True
Items 28 and 29, although often found in schizophrenia, carry much less diagnostic weight than the 'first-rank' symptoms.

31:True 32:False 33:False 34:True
Group therapy is as effective as individual psychotherapy. The prognosis is better than for anorexia nervosa.

35:True 36:True 37:True 38:True 39:True
Most significant medical illnesses can cause confusion, particularly in the elderly where cerebral reserve may be low. It occurs more commonly in association with any form of brain damage, anxiety, understimulation and drug dependence. Hypothyroidism can cause many of the commonest psychiatric syndromes i.e. acute confusion, dementia, depression and paranoid psychosis.

40:True 41:True 42:True 43:True 44:True
Physical harm or serious neglect of children tends to occur in parents with one or more of these characteristics: personality disorder, low social class, criminality, mental illness, marital disharmony and abuse in their own childhood. Certain features increase the risk of abuse: complications in pregnancy or labour, separation from mother in postnatal period, congenital defects and persistent crying.

45:False 46:False 47:False 48:True 49:False
The condition is twice as common in women as in men. There may be marked constitutional disturbance with fever, weight loss and anaemia. Treatment should be cautiously withdrawn as soon as there is clinical relief and a fall in the ESR.

50:True 51:False 52:False 53:True
The pain is characteristically relieved by sitting up and made worse by lying down. The traditional ECG finding of widespread raising of ST segments is actually uncommon and the ECG is rarely helpful.

54:False 55:False 56:True 57:True 58:False
There is no evidence of an autoimmune basis. About one third of all patients have a positive family history, but there is no regular Mendelian inheritance and only weak HLA associations. Some 70-80% of sufferers are non-smokers and giving up smoking may precipitate the first attack.

59:True 60:True 61:True 62:True 63:True
All are true. Radiotherapy involving irradiation of the bladder may cause fibrosis of the bladder wall and loss of normal visco-elasticity. Autonomic neuropathy due to diabetes or other causes may cause loss of bladder sensation.

64:True 65:False 66:True 67:True 68:True
The anaemia of chronic renal failure is normocytic or microcytic.

69:True 70:True 71:True 72:True 73:True
The systemic hypertension often seen in patients with obstructive sleep apnoea is poorly understood. Pulmonary hypertension and secondary polycythaemia are thought to result from the hypoxaemia that accompanies the episodes of apnoea, and which in some individuals may persist during waking hours. Daytime somnolence is characteristic; patients may fall asleep whilst driving, eating or talking. Depression affects at least 25% of patients.

74:True 75:True 76:True 77:True
A marked action tremor may run in families and is seldom suggestive of serious neurological disease. Action tremors, like many tremors, are worsened by anxiety. The drug of first choice for troublesome action tremors is propranolol but in patients in whom this drug is ineffective or contraindicated, low doses of primidone may be effective.

78:False 79:False 80:False 81:True 82:False
AIDS remains a clinical diagnosis and hence does not rely on serological tests for the Human Immunodeficiency Virus (HIV). Chest X-ray changes are similar for a variety of opportunistic infections and are not therefore diagnostic. There is at present no effective drug available to treat cryptosporidium. Encephalopathy and early dementia may result directly from HIV infection or from opportunists like cytomegalovirus. In the United Kingdom neither infection with HIV, nor the diagnosis of AIDS, are statutorily notifiable. However voluntary reporting of cases is encouraged to the Communicable Disease Surveillance Centre, where a confidential register is maintained.

83:True 84:False 85:True 86:False
Orthostatic proteinuria may accompany glomerular disease and is not necessarily benign.

87:True 88:False 89:True 90:False 91:True
Sexual maturation tends to be slightly delayed in diabetic children (especially in girls). There is no evidence of increased psychiatric morbidity. Microvascular disease is very uncommon in childhood but should never be ignored.

92:False 93:True 94:False 95:False 96:True
1-2% of school girls and 0.2% of boys have asymptomatic bacteriuria. In the first year of life the incidence is equal in boys and girls.

97:True 98:False 99:True 100:False 101:False
No distinct word at 18 months is one of the definitions of a late talker. Casting normally stops after 15 months. One year is the age of referral for not sitting alone.

102:True 103:False 104:True 105:True 106:False
Involvement of the antecubital and popliteal fossae is characteristic in older children and adults.

107:True 108:False 109:False 110:True 111:False
The patients are usually adults. In coloured subjects the lesions are hyperpigmented. Corticosteroids should be given until the itching subsides.

112:True 113:True 114:False 115:True 116:False
Iron deficiency may cause generalised pruritus, as may polycythaemia vera.

117:True 118:False 119:True 120:True 121:False
Tamoxifen is an anti-oestrogen and danazol inhibits the release of pituitary FSH and LH; both tend to reduce oestrogen stimulation of breast tissue and have been used in the treatment of mild gynaecomastia. Cyproterone acetate is an anti-androgen and removes androgenic inhibition of oestrogen stimulation. Any cytotoxic drug, but particularly the alkylating agents, may damage testicular tissue and so reduce androgen levels. Tricyclic antidepressants, phenothiazines and some other drugs occasionally cause gynaecomastia by unknown mechanisms.

122:True 123:False 124:False 125:True 126:True
Trimethoprim is a folic acid antagonist and hence macrocytic blood disorders can occur. Cotrimoxazole can cause both fever and Stevens-Johnson syndrome but these do not occur if trimethoprim is given alone. Diarrhoea is rare with both cotrimoxazole and trimethoprim.

127:True 128:True 129:True 130:False 131:False
Cholestyramine and rifampicin reduce the effect of warfarin and the dose would need to be increased.

132:True 133:True 134:False 135:True 136:False
Congenital abnormalities occur in 7% of babies born to epileptic mothers. Sodium valproate increases the risk of spina bifida to 1-2% (0.023% of all births). The incidence of congenital heart disease in the babies of mothers using phenytoin is 8%, it is also associated with orofacial clefts. Carbamazepine appears to be relatively safe, it is chloramphenicol which causes bone marrow supression. Warfarin is associated with c.n.s. defects, heparin is not implicated.

137:True 138:True 139:False 140:False 141:True
Ethanol not only reduces milk secretion but also sedates the infant. Metoclopramide increases milk production. Lithium does not affect the quantity of milk but causes hypotonia, hypothermia and cyanosis and is contra-indicated. Aspirin does not reduce milk but may cause a rash and impaired platelet function. Bromocriptine is very effective at supressing lactation.

142:False 143:False 144:True 145:False
Cigarette smoking is associated with an early menopause, presumably due to lower circulating oestrogen levels. The psychological symptoms often appear before flushes or vaginal dryness. Myocardial infarction is a relative contra-indication to HRT.

146:True 147:False 148:True
Oral contraception may decrease vaginal discharge, and this may predispose to skin trauma and thrush. Trichomonas is associated with a green frothy discharge.

149:True 150:False 151:True 152:False
It may cause renal damage and liver failure. It is not associated with fetal abnormality.

153:False 154:True 155:True 156:False 157:True
About 6% of pregnant women have asymptomatic bacteriuria which is defined as more than 100 000 organisms per ml in fresh urine. Bacteriuria is more common in lower social classes, and this may account for the association of anaemia and low birth weight with it.

158:True   159:True   160:False   161:False
Diabetes in pregnancy is associated with hypertension, hydramnios, increases in congenital abnormalities, intra-uterine death, large baby and various neonatal complications. There may be more rapid progression of retinopathy.

162:True   163:False   164:False   165:True
The pain of median nerve compression may radiate to the forearm and shoulder. Exacerbation by raising CSF pressure on coughing suggests nerve root compression in the neck.

166:False   167:True   168:True   169:False   170:True
RA is usually improved during pregnancy due to the increase of pregnancy-associated globulin which has anti-inflammatory properties. Dry mouth is a component of Sjogren's or sicca syndrome which occurs in many patients with RA. Sacroiliitis is not a feature of RA. Leg ulcers which are slow-healing are common.

171:True   172:False   173:False   174:True   175:False
The incubation periods are: diphtheria, 2-5 days; mumps, 12-21 days; rubella, 14-21 days; scarlet fever, 1-3 days; malaria, 10-14 days.

176:True   177:False   178:True   179:False   180:True
Presbyacusis is a loss of pure tone hearing in the higher frequencies. It is accompanied in about half of cases with abnormal loudness perception. Tinnitus is not necessarily associated with hearing loss. Two hearing aids (one in each ear!) are often better than one.

181:False   182:True   183:False   184:True
Diagnosis in the 60s or 70s reduces life expectancy to 65% of normal. Retinopathy is a late complication, so is uncommon in the elderly.

185:False   186:True   187:True   188:False   189:True
The incidence is 5% in over 65s. Loss of vision may occur quickly or very gradually. Halos and blurring may occur. The pupil is large on examination. A number of drugs are responsible for precipitating glaucoma.

190:False 191:False 192:False 193:True
The FHSA must be informed by the doctor with whom the patient is registered. No reason need be given. The patient is removed as soon as he/she joins another practice or 8 days later, whichever is the sooner.

194:False 195:True 196:True 197:True
Full time principals will normally be available for 42 weeks in any period of 12 months. GPs may also be available for 4 days if they are involved in organisation of the medical profession, training its members. Hours of availability do not include time on call or in practice administration.

198:True 199:False 200:True 201:True 202:True
A practice must provide a practice leaflet, and the items to be included are stipulated in the Terms of Service.

203:True 204:False 205:False 206:True 207:True
The Department of Health stated in 1990 that the FHSA should facilitate and monitor audit by setting up an independent group, which reports to FHSA. The groups dealings with individual GPs are confidential. They may use their resourses in a variety of ways to facilitate audit.

208:True 209:False 210:False
For contraception only form FP1003 should be completed. If you treat a patient you do not want to accept on your list you should complete an immediately necessary treatment form. The emergency treatment form is used if you have to attend a patient in an emergency who is not on your list. The UK has a reciprocal agreement with all EC countries and certain others to provide health care, and you will receive payment.

211:True 212:True 213:False 214:True
The general legislation applies to all employees but a written policy statement must be provided by employers of 5 staff. However if 4 people or less are present at any one time then the employer is exempted.

215:True 216:True 217:False 218:False 219:False
Associations include blood group A, male sex, low socio-economic group and smoking. Predisposing causes include achlorhydria and pernicious anaemia, intestinal metaplasia and previous gastric surgery. An abdominal mass is palpable only in 33%. Surgery is the treatment of choice, but most

have lymph node involvement at the time of surgery. Thus 5 year survival is usually less than 10%.

220:False 221:False 222:True 223:True
The death rate per year is over 30,000. 40% of primary tumours are squamous cell, 15% are adenocarcinomas.

224:True 225:True 226:False 227:False
The lack of investigation may give statistical errors. IHD is higher in soft water areas. It causes 25-30% of deaths in most western countries.

228:True 229:True 230:True 231:True 232:True
All should be taken as indications of serious intent. A suicide note would be a further sign of this.

233:True 234:True 235:False 236:False 237:True
The symptoms of agoraphobia include physical symptoms of anxiety; depersonalisation and avoidance of certain situations notably crowds, shops and transport. Aversion therapy is used to extinguish unwanted behaviour. In agoraphobia, the aim is to encourage certain behaviours in controlled conditions; the preferred behavioural treatment is programmed practice.

238:False 239:False 240:False 241:False 242:False
Patients with Munchausen's syndrome (hospital addiction) are classically males who fabricate physical and mental symptoms to obtain hospitalisation and treatment. They are evasive about their past and have psychopathic personality traits. They do not really believe themselves to be ill (unlike patients with hysteria). Prognosis is probably poor and many have repeated operations.

243:True 244:True 245:False 246:True 247:True
The most common effect of hypothyroidism on the menses is to cause menorrhagia, but other changes can occur. Anaemia may be normochromic or macrocytic.

248:True 249:True 250:True 251:True
All are correct.

252:True 253:True 254:False 255:True 256:True
A fall in plasma urate from a previously high level can precipitate acute gout, e.g. following administration of salicylates.

257:True 258:False 259:True 260:True
Hepatitis A virus may occasionally be shed during this period. Bed rest is unnecessary.

261:True 262:False 263:True 264:True
Therapy must continue for the rest of the patient's life.

265:True 266:False 267:True 268:False 269:True
The condition is mainly seen in adults. Although the ventricles are enlarged, the pressure within them is not persistently raised and papilloedema is absent. However, CSF diversion sometimes leads to improvement.

270:True 271:True 272:True 273:False 274:False
The guidelines are those of the British Thoracic Society. High doses of inhaled steroid should be continued in patients receiving oral maintenance steroids. Retention of CO_2 is not aggravated by treatment with oxygen in patients with severe acute asthma, the highest concentration available should be used.

275:True 276:False 277:True 278:True 279:True
Low birth weight and reduced growth rate in the first year are usual. All the other findings are recognised manifestations of the syndrome.

280:False 281:True 282:False 283:False 284:True
The absence of the Moro reflex is usually of serious significance, and occurs in kernicterus. There are usually 3 vessels in the umbilical cord, 2 may be a sign of renal abnormality. Umbilical hernias usually close spontaneously in the first year of life. Surgery may be indicated if still present at 2 years.

285:False 286:False 287:False 288:True 289:False
The condition is more common in women. Sunshine is an important precipitating factor, as is the incorrect use of topical corticosteroids. The condition is chronic and often persists for months or years if untreated.

290:False 291:True 292:True 293:True 294:True
They are the usual first line treatment in the obese. They interact with very few drugs as they are not protein bound and are excreted unchanged, however reduced renal clearance has been reported with cimetidine. They are rarely responsible for hypoglycaemic episodes. They should only be given to patients with normal renal function because of the risk of lactic acidosis. A metallic taste can occur without alcohol but is exacerbated by concurrent use.

295:False 296:False 297:False 298:False 299:False
There is no relationship between the tolerance to adverse and to therapeutic effects. Tolerance may develop in less than 48 hours after the initiation of treatment but is rapidly abolished once there is a nitrate free period. There is no difference between the various preparations. What is important is the length of time above the therapeutic level likely to cause tolerance in any one particular patient.

300:True 301:False 302:False 303:False 304:True
Absorption of drugs from the gut is influenced by many factors. If a drug is fat soluble the absorption will generally be enhanced in the presence of a fatty meal. Water soluble drugs such as digoxin and penicillin are best given with a drink of water one hour before a meal. The other three drugs are all gastric irritants and should be given with food.

305:True 306:False 307:True 308:False
The first attack is usually relatively severe and recurrences milder. Acyclovir is effective in shortening the attack.

309:False 310:True 311:True 312:True 313:False
PMT is not related to neuroticism, but may be worse at times of stress. Various dietary measures may help by diuretic action, increasing potassium and helping prevent carbohydrate craving. Up to 90% of women report symptoms at some time.

314:False 315:False 316:False 317:True
The patient should be investigated for iron, B12 and red cell folate levels. A bone marrow test is not required. Oral iron with folate will usually be sufficient, and transfusions or infusions should be avoided if possible.

318:False 319:False 320:True 321:True 322:True
Distinction must be made between *Salmonella* gastroenteritis, in which antibiotics are ineffective and the systemic forms of salmonellosis, (typhoid and paratyphoid) in which antibiotic therapy is essential. *Shigella sonnei* usually produces only mild diarrhoea and antibiotics are unnecessary.

323:False 324:False 325:True 326:True 327:True
TIA is defined as a focal loss of cerebral function from which full recovery occurs within 24 hours. Carotid TIAs have a worse prognosis as one third of patients will suffer stroke within 3 years. Hence endarterectomy should be considered.

328:True 329:False 330:False 331:True
Hypnotic benzodiazepines tend to cause an increase in REM sleep and therefore cause an increase in dreaming. Ataxia is very common in older patients and is the most important reason for limiting prescribing. There is no evidence that either osteomalacia or hypothermia are associated with prescribing of this drug.

332:True 333:False 334:False 335:True
Traumatic or inflammatory cataracts may develop more rapidly. Early referral is useful to allow the ophthalmologist to view the retina and see if it is healthy. Follow up can then be continued by the GP or optician until visual acuity deteriorates. Even when a cataract is advanced light and shadows are perceived.

336:True 337:True 338:False 339:True 340:True
The aims of treatment are to improve visual acuity in the squinting eye, improve appearance, and thirdly achieve binocular vision. The last aim is not achieved in the majority of cases, and children adapt and compensate well without, unlike adults. A child who tilts his head may be compensating for a vertical squint.

341:True 342:False 343:False
Examination must include height, weight and blood pressure. A fee may be claimed for consultations within 3 months of registering, and possibly up to 12 months if a special reason for its delay exists.

344:True 345:True 346:True 347:False
If the patient later provides evidence of being on the list the fee is returned. In road traffic accidents the account is submitted to the driver who can reclaim it from his/her insurance company.

348:False 349:False 350:False 351:False 352:False
The age range is 25-64. To reach the target 80% of eligible women should have been smeared, you are paid for the proportion of women who have been smeared by your own practice or a previous GP. The FHSA require the numbers of hysterectomised patients, but you need not submit a list, although one must be kept in the surgery.

353:False 354:False 355:True 356:True
Patients may see health records made since the 1st November 1991. A set charge may be made if the notes were not amended within 40 days of the application, or for photocopying or postage. If the correction is not thought necessary, a note of the applicants comments must be made at the appropriate point in the records.

357:True 358:True 359:False 360:True
The requirement regarding disabled people is on the understanding that suitable work is available. An employer is required to give an employee at least one weeks notice if employed continuously for 1 month for 16 or more hours per week. Employers must display an employer's liability certificate of insurance.

ANSWERS TO THE MEQ PAPER 1

A good candidate would be expected to:

1 • Establish a rapport and reason for current contact.
  • Establish baseline data of current and past medical history, drugs and allergies.
  • Develop preventative data, including date of last cervical smear and immunisation for tetanus.
  • Be aware of new patient check data requirements, including blood pressure, height, weight and urinalysis.
  • Share practice details with use of practice leaflet.
  • Assess current medical needs, based on baseline history and examination.
  • Share management plan of current and potential health problems.

2 • Establish a rapport with Tom and his mother.
  • Include Tom in decision making.
  • Explain the normal maturation process.
  • Take history and examination to determine primary or secondary enuresis — consider checking MSU.
  • Be aware of underlying psychological and social problems as contributory factors, including school and siblings.
  • Acknowledge short term imminent problem with appropriate treatment e.g. Imipramine or Desmopressin.
  • Make a joint management plan, recognising risk/benefit ratio of side effects.
  • Consider involvement of school, and confidentiality issues.
  • Appreciate long term management plan, with bell and mattress or other behavioural techniques.
  • Be aware of long-term family therapy.
  • Consider referral e.g. child psychologist, health visitor, paediatrician.

3 • Be aware of factors influencing compliance, including side effects of drugs, convenience of dosage, understanding of disease and rationale for drug use.
 • Appreciate financial factors, e.g. inability to afford prescription.
 • Be aware of psychological reactions to new illness, including rejection of diagnosis (and treatment) and depression and anxiety.
 • Possibility of incorrect diagnosis.
 • Angina deteriorating despite drug therapy.

4 • Be aware of Susan's rights and autonomy.
 • Appreciate highly emotional beginning to consultation and how this needs to be handled.
 • Establish whether both Susan and her mother wish to continue the consultation together or separately.
 • Options are:
    Continue joint consultation.
    Ask mother to leave the room and continue consultation with Susan.
    Suggest mother and Susan seen separately.
    Consider referral to another partner or health visitor/practice nurse.

5 • Establish 'why now'.
 • Allow Mr Partridge to express his concerns and worries, including exploration of underlying feelings of anger, guilt and anxiety.
 • Discuss present support systems including district nursing, health visiting, home help and meals on wheels.
 • Establish if requires greater input to support systems at home.
 • Consider personal coping mechanisms e.g. hobbies, leisure activities, support from friends, neighbours and relatives.
 • Establish if able to alleviate short term problems e.g. by FM3 certification or respite in hospital.
 • Appreciate stress of carers, show empathy and emphasise normality of their feelings.
 • Help Mr Partridge to consider pros and cons of retirement, in psychological, social and financial terms.

- Appreciate 'call for help' nature of presentation and possibility of medical or psychiatric problems in Mr Partridge.
- Establish how far he has already made enquiries into retirement. He may be wanting to reinforce a decision he has already made.
- Establish views on retirement held by wife, relatives, other carers and employer.
- Realise Mr Partridge's vulnerability.
- Discuss with primary health care team and arrange follow-up.

6 • Be aware of time constraints, for doctor, patient and waiting patients.
- Consider patient's autonomy and right to select agenda for consultation.
- Be aware of 'hidden agenda' with possibility of hidden fears, underlying problems, choice of this type of consultation as a defence mechanism.
- Appreciate the doctor's need to control the agenda of the consultation, to prioritise problems and also to keep to pre-planned consultation time.
- Be aware of doctor's feelings, including anger and anxiety.
- Be aware of the effect on the doctor of this consultation influencing subsequent consultations.
- Concern for possible missing of underlying pathology and connections between presentations.
- Be aware of ethical dilemmas of prescribing for absent patients.
- Consider modification of help-seeking behaviour pattern.
- Need to prioritise this session, with requirements for further consultations, possibly extended in time.
- Appreciate limited tasks achievable in one session e.g. need for patient education regarding HRT has to be postponed to another session.

7 • Establish if diabetic by performing blood sugar.
- Appreciate patient's worries and concerns (especially since asymptomatic) also knowledge of diabetes.
- Explain nature and management of diabetes.
- Consider medical management of diabetes, including possibility of referral.

- Be aware of role of practice nurse, and delegation of management, using practice protocols.
- Be aware of need to modify associated lifestyle factors, notably obesity and smoking.
- Advise patient to notify DVLA and car insurance company.
- Consider short and long term effect on work and family and appreciation of involving family.
- Obtain baseline investigations to establish end organ damage e.g. eyes and renal function.
- Appreciate need to involve patients in decisions and management.

8
- Appreciate that the wife is taking responsibility for husband's problems.
- Be aware of difficulties in husband/wife communication — both in initial discussion of problem and subsequent involvement in management.
- Only one party being privy to information, leading to possible distortion.
- Possible difficulties in getting husband to co-operate in recognising that he has a problem, and in reducing his intake.
- The fact that the husband does not as yet 'own' his problem.
- Establish 'why now'.
- Possibility of underlying recent problems within Mrs Morton (e.g. violence against her), or concern regarding Mr Morton's present physical or mental state.
- Presentation of hidden agenda, with possibility of presentation of Mrs Morton's own problems, either psychological, medical or social.
- Appreciate limited success in the consultation due to lack of patient.
- Possible breach of confidentiality if Mr Morton also one of your patients.

9
- Establish rapport and allow time for patient to express feelings e.g. guilt and anxiety.
- Develop trust to allow patient to state underlying concerns and worries.

- Be aware of patient's view of problems and their management.
- Appreciate problems in physical, psychological and social terms.
- Take appropriate history and examination.
- Establish present coping strategies and social support systems.
- Encourage utilisation of these.
- Appreciate underlying suicidal risk and take appropriate history.
- Consider referral e.g. health visitor or psychiatrist.
- Be aware of limited available time for consultation.
- Consider follow-up and sensitive ending to the consultation.
- Appreciate the effect on doctor's own feelings and allow time to recover if necessary prior to next consultation.

10 • Appreciate normality of emotions, including guilt, anger and sadness.
- Be aware of effect of emotional turmoil on personal and professional activities.
- Consider postponing on-call or making of major decisions.
- Reinforce personal strengths, both personal and professional.
- Appreciate variety of 'talking' resources e.g. spouse, partners, young principals group.
- Be aware of doctor's reluctance to approach professional helpers e.g. counsellor or psychiatrist.
- Appreciate importance of expressing emotions and effect of unexpressed emotion e.g. short-tempered or depressed.
- Be aware of 'short term comforts' (e.g. alcohol), with long term effects.

ANSWERS TO THE MEQ PAPER 2

A good candidate would be expected to:

1 • Consider 'why now'.
  • Establish rapport and empathise with Nancy on effect of sleeping difficulties on family.
  • Appreciate that probably at end of tether.
  • Determine Nancy's ideas, concerns and health beliefs on sleeping difficulties in young children.
  • Take detailed history (with particular emphasis on development of sleeping pattern) and examine to exclude painful conditions.
  • Be aware of underlying psychological and social factors in family.
  • Appreciate 'hidden agenda' — child as presenting complaint, of underlying medical, psychological and social problems for Nancy.
  • Consider effect of outside family influence e.g. mother and neighbours.
  • Explain normality of sleeping disturbance in young children and of behavioural principles.
  • Establish contract of short term rescue therapy rather than long term prescribing.
  • Involve Nancy in joint management plan.
  • Discuss risks and side-effects of sedatives versus benefits.
  • Consider extra support e.g. health visitor and referral e.g. child psychologist.
  • Arrange for follow-up.

2 • Appreciate the reasons for dissatisfaction with other doctor e.g.
      - difficulty with appointments
      - change in access e.g. altered bus route or car parking
      - clinical e.g. wrong diagnosis or treatment
      - staff e.g. partner, receptionist and nurses.
  • Altered expectations of health care including physical, psychological and social change.
  • Bad experience at last doctor — 'why now'.
  • Realise ease of change of doctor under new contract.
  • Change of doctor previously contemplated.

- Be aware of selection of your practice on positive grounds, following prompt from others e.g. nurse, family and neighbours.
- 'Hidden agenda' — wish to manipulate new doctor.

3 • Appreciate that patient anxious, thus need to establish good rapport.
- Acknowledge this anxiety.
- Be aware that patient already has ideas and concerns regarding diagnosis and X-ray result.
- Allow to voice these and build up information on diagnosis and result.
- Ensure setting appropriate for giving bad news e.g. quiet and uninterrupted, and also to make patient aware that you are going to discuss something important.
- Be aware of possible emotional responses to bad news e.g. denial, disbelief, anger.
- Consider possibility of having husband or family present.
- Give factual explanation of findings using simple non-technical language.
- Appreciate need to pace questioning. Allow patient to ask for information. Ensure information understood before proceeding further.
- Be aware of referral for further management and that patient will have to tolerate period of uncertainty until final diagnosis given.
- Consider management of present symptoms such as chronic cough.
- Review any medication.
- Arrange for follow-up and opportunity to discuss any further worries and concerns.
- Appreciate own feelings produced and need to handle these, especially before next patient.

4 • Be aware of literature available, including charts e.g. 'Pulse' or 'MIMS', British National Formulary, DHSS leaflet 'Advice To Travellers' SA40.
- Be aware of variety of information sources including local travel clinics e.g. Thomas Cook and British Airways, Hospitals for

Tropical Diseases, Hospitals for Communicable Diseases, pharmaceutical company databases.
- Appreciate information via Prestel, embassies and travel tour operators.
- Appreciate a wide variety of sources and possible difficulty in making definitive decisions on advice.

5 • Establish rapport and show empathy with her difficulties.
- Allow her to express any feelings e.g. anger, sadness.
- Consider 'why now'.
- Appreciate that it may be an acute problem that has precipitated her call for help.
- Consider appropriate management plan e.g. attend to medical, psychological and social problems.
- Acknowledge Mrs Richards' ideas and concerns regarding the future management.
- Consider if hospital appropriate.
- Appreciate mother-in-law's autonomy in making decision, although possibly she has no insight into her present situation.
- Be aware of risk versus benefit balance of long term hospital care against residential social services care.
- Recognise need to assess mother-in-law to confirm stated condition and decide on appropriate referral, whether medical or psychiatric.
- Appreciate need to offer continuing support to Mrs Richards and her family. Take detailed history, including drugs taken to establish if precipitating cause.
- Appreciate that other family members need to be involved in the decision i.e. son and other children.

6 • Acknowledge patients' confusion, about family therapy and also about Steven's illness.
- Consider hidden agenda e.g. wanting to discuss Steven and his illness and its management and their thoughts on therapy.
- Appreciate parents' ideas, beliefs and concerns regarding family therapy.
- Discuss what has already been stated by psychiatrist since this may have been misunderstood.

- Provide information on family therapy.
- Be aware of principles of giving information i.e. in small amounts, non-technical, simple explanations based on information requested, checking for understanding and opportunity to ask questions.
- Consider parents' feelings of guilt or blame for Steven's illness.
- Appreciate role of family as a unit and that changing one member affects other members.

7
- Maintain good relationships with both Tessa and health visitor.
- Encourage good rapport between Tessa and health visitor.
- Appreciate difficult boundary of allowing autonomy for Tessa but also concern for Paula.
- Establish ideas, concerns and feelings for Paula from both Tessa and health visitor.
- Acknowledge role of doctor in establishing diagnosis of 'failure to thrive' and decision on further investigation and referral.
- Be aware of variety of factors producing 'failure to thrive', medical, psychological and social.
- Take full history, examination and use of sequential weights on percentile charts.
- Establish shared management plan, involving Tessa and health visitor in management decisions.
- Consider necessity for follow-up.
- Consider possibility of family 'at risk' and discuss with other partners.

8 Appreciate complex combination of physical, psychological and social factors affecting Tessa's behaviour.
a) Medical e.g. underlying physical illness such as anaemia or glandular fever.
b) Psychological e.g. underlying depression, low IQ, not appreciating importance of adequate diet or effect of drug taking — medical or illicit.
c) Social e.g. poor mother/child bonding, factors affecting food purchase and preparation e.g. low income with inadequate kitchen facilities.

- Be aware of effect of being de-skilled by dominant health visitor or own mother, leading to apathy.

9
- Be aware of difficult boundaries between duties to patient and to society.
- Appreciate duty to patient, notably confidentiality regarding burglary and taking illegal drugs.
- Appreciate responsibility to society and where the boundary of disclosure is.
- Consider management of underlying addiction problems and any associated medical problems.
- Consider constraints on note keeping in patient's medical record.
- Appreciate legal obligation to notify addict to Home Office Drugs Branch.
- Be aware that patient has a significant habit and is willing to resort to violence, and theft.
- Have concern for own safety and practice security and the effect of this on the doctor-patient relationship.
- Consider possible hepatitis/HIV infection risk of open wound and possible duty of notifying nursing staff if requires dressing.
- Be aware of ethical dilemma of possible breaking of confidentiality to protect staff.

10
- Consider recognition of at-risk groups such as indices of deprivation e.g. Jarman index.
- Establish practice profile of amount of social deprivation in practice.
- Develop awareness of various problems in socially deprived areas and the complex mix of medical, psychological and social problems.
- Be aware of importance of team approach with good liaison between health visitors and social workers.
- Realize importance of good working relationships and multidisciplinary communication about problems and areas of responsibility.
- Appreciate difficulties in access to medical care, and in developing a responsive service.

- Consider staff training to enable understanding of particular problems.
- Be aware of importance of other agencies involved in social care e.g. housing departments and voluntary agencies.
- Appreciate importance of developing effective practice policies for delivery of all care, medical and also preventive e.g. immunisation.

ANSWERS TO THE CRQ PAPERS

Sample CRQ Paper : Question 1A.

Can Health Screening Damage Your Health?

1. Summarise the article attached.

Objective. To determine if screening may make participants with no risk factors for the disease more aware of illness, thus increasing their psychological distress.

Design. A prospective randomised cohort study using questionnaires.

Setting. Suburban British general practice.

Patients. For the study group all attenders, selected from age/sex register, at a coronary risk screening clinic and, for the control group, a random sample of non-invited patients similarly matched for age.

Main outcome measures. Use of the 30 item General Health Questionnaire (GHQ) as an indicator of psychological wellbeing.

Results. 215 patients in study group, with 225 controls. Comparing GHQ scores, significantly fewer of those attending for screening had psychological distress than the control group at the initial questionnaire but at the second questionnaire three months later the screened group had a significantly higher GHQ score. The control group had a non-significant fall in GHQ score over the same 3 month period.

Conclusion. The initial hypothesis, in the objective of the study, was supported.

2. Comment on the design of the study and the presentation of the results.

a) Good points
- Achievable stated objective that was followed throughout the study.
- Controlled study — prospective better than retrospective.
- Good selection of control groups, well matched to study group for age, sex and social class variables.
- Good randomisation.
- Use of standard assessment tool for psychological distress i.e. 30 item GHQ.
- Follow up of non-responders after 10 days.
- Study of interest to all GPs.

- Numbers in study appear to be adequate.
- Clearly presented results and data.

b) Bad points
- The control group had a poor completion, with only 68.8% completing the first and second questionnaire whereas the screen group was 87.9%.
- Accompanying letter to control group could have been alarmist.
- Unexpected results, for both control and study groups which were apparently inexplicable.
- Study group shows increase over 3 months of psychological distress but control group shows fall. Explanations of this appear to be 'dredged' from other studies.
- Sole indicator of psychological distress was the GHQ.
- How relevant compared with other measures?
- Does not look at screen group who had risk factors of cardiovascular disease detected.
- Applicable to other screening?

3. If the conclusions of this paper were supported by further research, what are the implications for you as a general practitioner?

- Increase in consultations — the 'worried well'.
- Questions whether other screening produces similar adverse effects.
- Helps us to question what we feel we are doing well but has not been proven.
- Questions our whole approach to health screening, e.g. what information we give the patient in the letter of introduction.
- Makes us aware of increased stress that patients may suffer as a result of increased cardiovascular system screening.
- Shakes the assumption of all screening, i.e. not to cause harm to the asymptomatic.

Sample CRQ Paper : Question 1B.

GPs advice for travellers to Turkey

1. **Summarise the article attached.**

   Objective – to determine the advice given by general practitioners (including immunisation, prophylactic medication and other advice) to a young man travelling to Turkey and their own resources of guidance for this information.

   Design – a postal survey using a questionnaire in which a clinical scenario is presented and questions of intended action are asked.

   Setting – principals in general practice in Inverclyde, Scotland.

   Subjects – details obtained from 50 principals.

   Main outcome measures –
   1. Listing recommended immunisations and prophylactic medication.
   2. Other advice given regarding trip to Turkey.
   3. Whether consulted for travel advice to Turkey in the year prior to the study.
   4. Whether doctor had visited Turkey himself.

   Results - there was an 83% response rate and 82% had been consulted by a prospective traveller to Turkey in the previous year and 10% of the GPs had visited Turkey themselves. 96% would recommend typhoid, 78% cholera and 74% polio immunisation, all of which are recommended by the DHSS in leaflet SA40. 52% recommend antimalarials, although SA40 is ambiguous. Advice not recommended in SA40 included tetanus immunisation given by 40% and human normal immunoglobulin given by 12%. There was a wide variety of sources of information, the most popular being weekly medical newspapers. Other advice to travellers included care with food given by 70%, risks of excessive sun exposure given by 50% and advice on 'safe sex' given by 18%.

   Conclusion - there is wide variety in both advice given and the sources of such advice. Only 36% gave advice as detailed in SA40, which was only referred to as a source of information by 4% of respondents.

2. **Comment on the design of the study and the presentation of the results.**

   a) Good points
   - Good response to questionnaire (83%).

- Sent to 60 out of 62 principals in one health district.
- Good follow-up of non-responders.
- Good statistics and clear presentation in tables.
- Clinically relevant to all GPs.

b) Bad points
- Sufficient number of respondents?
- Excluded advice by practice nurses.
- Excluded other definitive sources of information e.g. Public Health Laboratory Service, Hospital for Tropical Diseases and Prestel.
- Based on stated intention not actual observed behaviour.
- Clinical scenario may not reflect true management with actual patient.
- No pilot of questionnaire stated.

3. **If the conclusions of this paper were supported by further research, what are the implications for you as a general practitioner?**

- Awareness of conflicting advice and wide variety of sources of information.
- Difficulty of adequate delegation to practice nurse to give advice.
- Difficulties in using and updating information systems available regarding travel advice.
- Concern that no consistent advice given to individual patients since different doctors use different sources of information.
- Increased prescribing costs due to unnecessary immunisation.

<u>Sample CRQ Paper : Question 3A.</u>

Practice Annual Report

1. **Comment on the above data.**
    - The candidate is expected to demonstrate the ability to extract information from a pie chart.
    - Doctor 1 has 202 hospital referrals, over twice that of doctor 5 (100) and also significantly higher than that of any other doctor in the practice. Doctor 2 is the next highest referrer with 177.
    - Appreciation of limitation of gross figures, without further information e.g. list size, part/full time partners etc.
    - Uncertainty of what it relates to e.g. is it in-patient, out-patient, which specialty and to which hospitals?

2. **What are the possible causes of variation in hospital referrals made by each doctor?**
    - Appreciation of wide variety of hospital referrals between individual doctors and that many factors involved.
    - Appreciation of difficulties when no further breakdown of information e.g. whether referred to in-patients or out-patients and which individual specialties. Also whether includes patient self referrals e.g. to casualty departments.
    - Appreciation of various factors involved:

    a) **patients** — the doctor may look after a particular group of patients with problems requiring referral e.g. elderly in nursing homes.

    b) **GP** — special interest e.g. increased referrals for certain specialist investigation. Poorer confidence when dealing with problems in a general practice setting. Different personal list sizes, including whether trainer and trainee referrals added to responsible partner's figures. Availability e.g. part-time partners or holidays and sick/maternity leave during the study period.

Sample CRQ Paper : Question 3B.

Doctor's Letter

1. What issues are raised?
- Patient autonomy and right to choose
- Continuity of care
- GP as patient's advocate
- Transfer from private care to NHS list during treatment
- Private care as initial contact to by-pass long NHS waiting list
- Consultant accepting patient by direct referral rather than through GP

2. List the advantages and disadvantages of open referral.

Patient
Advantages:
Quicker access to specialist care.
No need to bother GP, especially if poor doctor-patient relationship.
Perceived satisfaction that seeing a specialist rather than a generalist.

Disadvantages:
May choose inappropriate specialist for problem.
May lead to inappropriate management and investigations.

Doctor (GP)
Advantages: allows more time with other patients.

Disadvantages: lack of continuity of care.

Consultant Ophthalmologist
Advantage: easier access and shorter waiting time for appointment.

Disadvantage: no background information, leading to increased and duplicated investigations.

Optician
Advantage: promotes autonomy by direct referral to consultant.

Disadvantage: not aware of significant past medical history or other background information.

Society e.g. private insurance company or NHS
Advantages: general perceived increased satisfaction of quick and easy access to a specialist opinion.

Disadvantages: could be more expensive since no initial pre-selection and advice regarding referral.

Sample CRQ Paper : Question 3C.

Asthma Protocol

List recommendations for improving the asthma protocol giving your reasons.

- The purpose of the protocol should be defined and stated, also whether it applies to acute or chronic care and which age group it is to be used for.
- The protocol is disorganised and should be rewritten.
- The intended users of the protocol are not stated and should be agreed and stated.
- The word asthma should be highlighted clearly on patient records.
- Patients' access to immediate treatment should be easy.
- The use of peak flow meters in management and use of maintenance inhaled steroids should follow accepted management plan e.g. British Thoracic Society recommendations.
- Steroid usage should be clearly defined.
- The protocol should be capable of audit.
- The responsibility of individual team members should be clearly stated.
- The use of nebulisers and their limitation should be more clearly defined.

MEDICAL AUDIT

One of the current areas of interest in general practice, both within the profession (via the RCGP and the GMSC) and the DHSS (via the FHSA) is medical audit. This has been defined as 'the systematic critical analysis of the quality of medical care, including the procedures used for diagnosis and treatment, the use of resources and the resulting outcome and quality of care of life for the patient.' Department of Health, January 1989.

Medical audit can be seen as a series of steps (The Audit Cycle).

Step 1.   Choose a topic and set a standard.
Step 2.   Compare present practice with this standard.
Step 3.   Modify your practice to make the standard attainable.
Step 4.   Repeat the process to confirm improvement.

Step 1. The choice of topic is vast. Involvement by all staff concerned is important, since their future commitment is paramount. Often a topic with financial implications e.g. immunisation targets or one in which clinical care has been questioned e.g. sudden death can be chosen. It should be relevant to the practice's needs and lead to improved patient care. The topic area can be chosen from several areas e.g.

(a) Practice structure e.g. surgery premises, range and type of equipment, the records system and organisational systems design.
(b) Processes e.g. examinations undertaken, prescriptions written, tests carried out, advice given.
(c) Outcomes e.g. social functioning, psychological functioning, physical functioning and patient satisfaction.

When conducting an audit a very specific question should be asked e.g. How good is our management of hypertension? An agreed standard is then determined e.g. 80% of patients with established hypertension aged 20-35 will have a diastolic less than 90 millimetres of mercury within the first year of treatment.

Step 2. Data should be collected so that it can be compared to the agreed standard.

Step 3. Collecting data is only of value if a change in practice occurs. The practice needs to be modified so that the agreed standard is reached. This involves team work and delegation.

Step 4. This is widely seen as the most important stage — often called 'closing the loop' since it demonstrates if improvement is actually being achieved.

The above principles apply to all aspects of medical audit. A knowledge of these concepts is expected from candidates as is their application to day to day practice. This aspect is looked for in the oral examination, especially in relation to the Practice Experience Questionnaire. A section for audit can be seen on looking at this paper. One method of preparation is to undertake a small simple audit in practice — the various difficulties will thus become readily apparent! Candidates are expected to know how medical audit is organised, e.g. via Medical Audit Advisory Groups.

Whenever change in practice needs to be implemented a knowledge of the process of management is required. Excellent introductions are available in *Making Sense of Audit* edited by Donald and Sally Irvine published by Radcliffe Medical Press Ltd and *Managing Change in Primary Care* by M Pringle et al, also published by Radcliffe Medical Press Ltd.

THE CONSULTATION

The consultation is the central task of general practice. Consultation skills form the basis of good patient care. It has been shown that consultation skills can be learnt and that to do so requires systematic training rather than just experience. Hence it is vital that you have an understanding of consultation models. You may be asked about consultations in the oral exam but you will also find the understanding of consultations helpful in the MEQ part of the paper.

Various models have been described to help explain what happens in a consultation. A summary of the various approaches used is given to allow an overall view of the subject.

1. **Description of Events Occurring in a Consultation (after Byrne and Long 1976)**

   This model was produced after analysing over 2,000 tape recordings of consultations. They identified six phases that form a logical structure to the consultation.

   1. The doctor establishes a relationship with the patient.

   2. The doctor either attempts to discover, or actually discovers, the reason for the patient's attendance.

   3. The doctor conducts a verbal or physical examination, or both.

   4. The doctor, or the doctor and the patient together, or the patient alone (usually in that order of probability) consider(s) the condition.

   5. The doctor, and occasionally the patient, details treatment or further investigation.

   6. The consultation is terminated — usually by the doctor.

2. Expansion to Include Preventative Care

In 1979 Stott and Davies described four areas which could be systematically explored each time a patient consults:

1. Management of presenting problems

2. Management of continuing problems

3. Modification of help-seeking behaviour

4. Opportunistic health promotion

3. A Model of Seven Tasks

This model was detailed by Pendleton et al in 1984. It lists seven tasks which form an effective consultation. The model emphasises the importance of the patient's view and understanding of the problem.

1. To define the reasons for the patient's attendance including:
   - The nature and history of the problem
   - Their cause
   - The patient's ideas, concerns and expectations
   - The effects of the problems

2. To consider other problems:
   - Continuing problems
   - Risk factors

3. To choose with the patient an appropriate action for each problem.

4. To achieve a shared understanding with the patient.

5. To involve the patient in the management plan and encourage him to accept appropriate responsibility.

6. To use time and resources appropriately.

7. To establish or maintain a relationship with the patient which helps to achieve the other tasks.

4. Health Belief Model

This model was devised by Rosenstock in 1966, and Becker and Maiman in 1975. It looks at the patient's reasons for accepting or rejecting the doctor's opinion. It shows that the patient is more likely to accept advice, diagnosis or treatment if the doctor is aware of their ideas, concerns and expectations.

It looks at various factors:

1. People vary in their interest in health — 'health motivation'.

2. Patients vary in how likely they think they are to contract an illness — 'perceived vulnerability'.

3. Patients' belief in the diagnosis is affected by whether they feel their opinion or 'concerns' have been understood by the doctor.

4. 'Perceived seriousness' varies between patients for a given condition.

5. Six Categories of Intervention

This was devised by a psychologist, John Heron, in the mid 1970s, as a model of interventions which can be used by the doctor.

1. Prescriptive: Instructions or advice — directive.

2. Informative: Explaining and giving information.

3. Confronting: Giving feedback to the patient on their behaviour or attitude, in order to help them see what is happening.

4. Cathartic: Helping the patient to release their emotions.

5. Catalytic: Encouraging the patient to explore his own feelings and reasons for behaviour.

6. Supportive: Encouraging the patient's self worth e.g. by giving approval.

6. Transactional Analysis

This model of communication was described by Eric Berne in the 1960s. It explores our behaviour within relationships. It identifies three 'ego-states' — Parent, Adult and Child — any one of which an individual could be experiencing at any time. It looks at the implications and reasons for the different states. It also explores 'games', which can be used to identify why transactions repeatedly go wrong.

This model is useful for exploring consultations by looking at the relationship between the doctor and the patient.

7. Balint

This work in the 50s explored the importance of the doctor-patient relationship. It explored the importance and identification of psychological problems. It suggested the following concepts:

1. 'The doctor as the drug.' The 'pharmacology' of the doctor as a treatment.

2. 'The child as the presenting complaint.' The patient may offer another person as the problem when there are underlying psycho-social problems.

3. 'Elimination by appropriate physical examination.' This may reinforce the patient's belief that his symptoms (neurotic in origin) are in fact due to physical illness. Repeated investigations perpetuate this cycle.

4. 'Collusion of anonymity.' As above, referral reinforces mistaken belief in the origin of symptoms. The responsibility of uncovering underlying psycho-social problems becomes increasingly diluted by repeated referral, with nobody taking final responsibility.

5. 'The Mutual Investment Company.' This is formed and managed by the doctor and the patient. 'Clinical illnesses' are episodes in a long relationship and represent 'offers' of problems (physical and psycho-social) to the doctor.

6. 'The flash.' The point in the consultation when the real reason of the 'offer' (underlying psycho-social and neurotic illness) is suddenly apparent to both doctor and patient. This forms a fulcrum for change; the consultation can now deal with the underlying basic 'fault'.

8. The Inner Consultation

This work by Roger Neighbour published in 1987 looks at improving consultation skills. He uses the following format for the consultation.

1. Connecting: Rapport building skills

2. Summarising: Listening and eliciting skills

3. Handover: Communicating skills

4. Safety netting: Predicting skills. Contingency plans of what and when further action may be needed.

5. Housekeeping: Taking care of yourself, checking you are ready for the next patient.

It is not suggested that you should memorise the above models, but you should have an understanding of at least some of them. You should also be aware of how you can analyse your own consultation methods — and how you could work on improving them i.e. use of video or audio tape recordings, simulated consultations with actors, role play or colleagues 'sitting in'.

APPENDIX 3

SAMPLE PRACTICE EXPERIENCE QUESTIONNAIRE (PEQ)

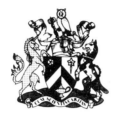

THE ROYAL COLLEGE OF GENERAL PRACTITIONERS

EXAMINATION FOR MEMBERSHIP

The oral examination will consist of two parts, each half-an-hour and each part being with a different pair of examiners.

The first oral will be devoted to examining the candidate using his/her Practice Experience Questionnaire as the basis for topics to consider. Although trainees and candidates from the Services may not have been able to influence the practices described, they will be expected to have a good working knowledge of the practice organisation, though not necessarily to justify it.

Part of the time will be spent on considering the practice, its facilities, organisation and services, and part on the clinical record. Candidates may bring to the examination brief clinical notes on the patients listed.

Candidates not in practice currently must complete the Clinical Diary and should describe a practice in which they have worked. If possible patients should have been managed recently in general practice, if necessary by undertaking some part-time or locum work.

The second oral will be based on topics arising from the presentation and management of clinical problems chosen by the examiners.

The candidate may also be asked to comment on issues relating to the profession in general and general practice in particular.

Candidates will be expected to satisfy the examiners that they can apply their knowledge and skills to total personal care in clinical, psychological and social terms.

Please note that there have been some alterations to the questionnaire (formerly called the Log Diary). These are partly to reflect the changes that have occurred in practice organisation recently, or are expected to result from the 1990 Contract; and partly (as in Sections E and F) to make the questionnaire more relevant to the candidate's own learning and clinical experiences.

PRACTICE EXPERIENCE QUESTIONNAIRE (LOG DIARY)

The information requested in this questionnaire will provide a basis for discussion in the first oral. It will not, in itself, attract any marks.

SECTION A. CANDIDATE'S PERSONAL DATA

1. Name: 2. Examination number

3. Address:

4. Your present status in general practice: (Please tick)

   Principal
   Assistant
   Trainee

5. Your total experience in general practice: Years
                                                      Months

6. Length of time in present post: Years
                                                      Months

SECTION B. PRACTICE STRUCTURE

7. Total list size:

   Percentage   Under 5   65-74   Over 75
   of patients

8. Premises and Practice Features: (Please tick)

   Purpose-built   Urban

   Converted   Rural

   Partnership-owned   Mixed

   Rented   Dispensing

   LHA Health Centre   Budget-holding

   Other   Undergraduate teaching

                              Training

9. Number of doctors providing General Medical Services:

   Partners full-time   Assistants

   Partners part-time   Trainees

10. Please comment on any special, social, ethnic or other features of the practice:

143

SECTION C. PRACTICE ORGANISATION AND FACILITIES

11. Staff. Please list the various categories of ancillary staff working in the practice and sho
the numbers in each category.

Nursing and Paramedical

Employed	part/full		Attached	part/full

Clerical and Administrative

Employed	part/full		Attached	part/full

12. Is Child Health Surveillance approved within the practice?   Yes/No

13. Is minor surgery approved within the practice?   Yes/No

14. What health promotion clinics are approved within the practice?

15. What additional clinics/sessions exist within the practice?
eg obstetrics, immunisation, screening?

16. What systems for audit exist within the practice?

17. What special diagnostic, therapeutic or other equipment is available within the Practice (eg ECG, sonicaid, autoclave)?

Diagnostic	Therapeutic and other

18. What diagnostic or therapeutic facilities are available by direct access outside the Practice (eg X-ray, ultrasound, endoscopy, physiotherapy)?

Diagnostic	Therapeutic

19. Is there a computer in the Practice?   Yes/No

    If so, what are its principal uses?

20. How are out-of-hours duties covered?   (Please tick)

    Rota within Practice   Rota with one other Practice
    Deputising Service   Rota with several Practices

SECTION D.   WORK LOAD ANALYSIS

21. Please state the numbers of patients seen in a recent typical week.

    a) by all doctors

	M	T	W	Th	F	S
consulting am						
consulting pm						
special surgeries or clinics						
new home visits						
repeat home visits						

    b) by the candidate

consulting am						
consulting pm						
special surgeries or clinics						
new home visits						
repeat home visits						

22. Does the Practice have access to
    a GP Obstetric Unit?   Yes/No

    How many confinements were   )   in complete care
    there in a recent quarter?   )   in shared care

23. What is the Practice's consulting rate
    (doctor-patient consultations per patient per year)?

SECTION E. CANDIDATE'S OWN IDEAS AND LEARNING EXPERIENCE

24. Describe two or three features of the Practice which you have found to be interesting or
    stimulating; or which have influenced your attitudes; or which have helped you improve
    your knowledge or skills; or an audit or study that you have carried out.

25. What changes would you suggest for the next three years to improve the Practice?

SECTION F.   CLINICAL DIARY

Please list the relevant numbers of patients seen consecutively in each of the following categories:- surgery attendances – 25 cases; home visits – 15 cases; out-of-hours emergencies – 10 cases including 2 night calls whenever possible. These cases will provide examples for examination of your clinical abilities. You may bring brief clinical notes about them to the examination.

No.	Date	Patient's Initials	Age	Sex	Main reason for contact
Surgery Attendances					
1.					
2.					
3.					
4.					
5.					
6.					
7.					
8.					
9.					
10.					
11.					
12.					
13.					
14.					
15.					
16.					
17.					
18.					
19.					
20.					
21.					
22.					
23.					
24.					
25.					

Appendix 3 : Sample Practice Experience Questionnaire

No.	Date	Patient's Initials	Age	Sex	Main reason for contact
Home Visits and repeat visits					
26.					
27.					
28.					
29.					
30.					
31.					
32.					
33.					
34.					
35.					
36.					
37.					
38.					
39.					
40.					

Out-of-hours and emergency calls. Indicate night visits "NV"

If sufficient cases in this category cannot be found please say why this is so.

41.					
42.					
43.					
44.					
45.					
46.					
47.					
48.					
49.					
50.					

PasTest Books and Intensive Revision Courses

Short Notes for the DCH

Joseph Blackburn MRCP MRCGP DRCOG DCH
Gerald Curtis Jenkins DRCOG FRCGP

This revision book for the Diploma in Child Health is designed for exam candidates and general practitioners. It covers the full syllabus including model answers for the Short Note questions and synopses of favourite Case Commentary and Clinical Exam topics. Chapters are arranged by specialty and by symptom, and a revision plan, MCQ topics and reading list are also included. No candidate should be without this book.
ISBN: 0 906896 703

The DRCOG Examination: A Structured Approach

Stuart Mellor MB ChB MRCOG
Michael Read MD FRCS MRCOG FRACOG
Stuart Bootle MB ChB DRCOG MRCGP
John Sandars MB ChB(hons) MRCP MRCGP

Written by a team of two examiners and two GPs, this book covers in detail the three parts of the DRCOG exam - written, clinical and oral. It offers advice on technique and a unique analysis of the exam. It also includes MCQs, teaching notes, model essays, clinical and oral exam advice, checklists, answering schedules and revision topics. This is an invaluable book for both candidates and trainers.
ISBN: 0 906896 614

For details on PasTest Intensive Courses P.T.O

PasTest Intensive Courses

- High quality professional courses
- Benefit from our 21 years experience in medical education
- Past College exam questions form the basis for all teaching sessions
- Approval under HM 67/27, Section 63 or PGEA

MRCGP Weekend Courses (London and Manchester)

These courses are run by RCGP examiners and are designed to cover all aspects of the exam: MCQs, MEQs, Critical Reasoning, revision planning, popular topics, oral video with working papers, analyses and discussion. Practice questions are forwarded for completion before the course.
Held in April and October each year.

DRCOG Weekend Courses (London and Manchester)

This course covers all parts of the syllabus in Obstetrics, Gynaecology, Family Planning and Paediatrics. Mock vivas and problem circuits will allow candidates to develop their knowledge and a revision checklist is provided. Practice questions are forwarded for completion before the course. Held in March and September each year.

DCH Weekend Courses (London and Manchester)

This intensive course covers all aspects of paediatrics needed for this diploma. The extensive lecture notes and handouts are based on past exam questions. Precourse material is provided.
Held in August and December each year.

Courses are also provided for MRCP Part 1, MRCP Part 2 (General Medicine and Paediatrics), and PLAB for overseas trained doctors.

For more details about PasTest books and courses please use the form opposite without delay.

REQUEST FORM

Please send me by return of post the information ticked below:

      Revision Books ☐

      MRCGP courses :   London ☐   Manchester ☐

      DCH courses   :   London ☐   Manchester ☐

      DRCOG courses :   London ☐   Manchester ☐

Name_____

Address_____

_____

Telephone_____

PasTest, Rankin House, Parkgate, Knutsford,
Cheshire WA16 8DX. Tel 0565 755226 Fax 0565 650264.

                                                      GPB

NOTES

NOTES